THE MEDICINE-FREE, ILLNESS-FREE SERIES

AMINO ACID THERAPY

Fueling Strength and Happiness with Amino Acids

Forest Yin, DAOM, L.Ac.

Ashi Healing Publishing

AF884371

Copyright © 2025 by Dr. Forest Yin

All rights reserved.

No part of this book may be reproduced, stored, or transmitted in any form or by any means—electronic, mechanical, photocopying, recording, or otherwise—without prior written permission from the publisher, except for brief quotes used in reviews.

First Edition: May 2025

Published by Ashi Healing

www.AshiHealing.com

Paperback ISBN: 978-1-967735-08-2

eBook ISBN: 978-1-967735-09-9

Printed in the United States of America

Medical Disclaimer:

This book is for informational purposes only and is not intended as medical advice. The author and publisher assume no responsibility for how the information is used. Readers should consult a healthcare professional before making any health-related decisions.

Foreword

Nature is the origin of life, the origin of healing, and remains a guiding force in human well-being. Long before modern science developed medicine in laboratories, nature provided everything the human body needed to survive, and to sustain life. The food we eat, the herbs we gather, the minerals beneath our feet, and the sun above us are all part of an intelligent and interconnected system that has long nourished and supported the human body.

This truth has been known across cultures for thousands of years, and it is echoed in sacred texts. In the Book of Genesis, the Garden of Eden was described as a paradise where "every tree that is pleasant to the sight and good for food" was made available to humankind (Genesis 2:9). Some scholars believe this refers not only to nourishment, but also to the ability to contribute to human well-being. It becomes even more clear in Ezekiel 47:12: "The fruit thereof shall be for meat, and the leaf thereof for medicine."

Somewhere along the way, modern culture drifted from this wisdom. Many now believe that healing must come through synthetic drugs, surgeries, or man-made interventions, forgetting that the foundation of human health has always been rooted in nature. But what if well-being isn't only about medical breakthroughs, but also about reconnecting with what has always been available to us?

What if the body doesn't need to be forced to function differently, but simply supported, nourished, balanced, and reminded of what it already knows? What if illness is not the enemy, but a signal that we've fallen out of balance, and out of sync with nature?

This is not to dismiss the value of conventional medicine. We are deeply grateful for its life-saving capabilities in emergencies and acute care. But when it comes to supporting long-term vitality and encouraging balance, it may be time to return to the source.

In addition to thousands of years of lived wisdom, modern science is now exploring the potential of many natural approaches. What was once viewed as "alternative" is now increasingly recognized as part of a broader wellness conversation.

This book, and the entire *Medicine-Free, Illness-Free Series,* is rooted in this truth: Nature not only gave us life. Many believe it holds the power to support our well-being. And many of these natural approaches are now being studied and better understood through science.

Healing is not something we must force or fear. It is something we can encourage, by gently supporting the body, naturally.

Dr. Forest Yin, DAOM, L.Ac.

Author, *The Medicine-Free, Illness-Free Series*

Founder, Ashi Healing and Acupuncture Inc.

Important Disclaimer

The supplements, therapies, and natural approaches discussed in *The Medicine-Free, Illness-Free Series* are intended to support general wellness and the body's natural balance. They are not intended to diagnose, treat, cure, or prevent any disease and have not been evaluated by the U.S. Food and Drug Administration (FDA).

These books are provided for educational purposes only and are not a substitute for professional medical advice, diagnosis, or treatment. Always consult your physician or a licensed healthcare provider before starting any new supplement, therapy, or wellness routine, especially if you are pregnant, nursing, have a medical condition, or are taking medications.

The content in this series is informed by two sources: summaries of available scientific research, presented as "Science-Informed Solution Benefits", and aggregated user feedback, presented as "Customer-Reported Solution Benefits". These are intended to inform and inspire, but they reflect general patterns, not guarantees. Individual results will vary.

The phrase *"Medicine-Free, Illness-Free"* reflects a natural wellness philosophy and is not a medical claim or promise of outcome.

By reading this book, you agree to take full responsibility for your personal health choices and to seek guidance from qualified health professionals when needed.

Contents

Preface

Do you feel like you've tried everything—medications, conventional treatments, even supplements—yet still struggle with fatigue, discomfort, brain fog, or other daily wellness concerns?

If so, you're not alone.

Many people today are turning to nature-based solutions, not as replacements for essential medical care, but as gentle, sustainable ways to support their overall well-being.

The rise in chronic health challenges reflects this shift. According to the CDC, over 60% of U.S. adults live with at least one chronic health condition, and more than 40% manage two or more. More than 40% of school-aged children in the United States are reported to have at least one ongoing wellness concern, rising sharply in recent years.

At the same time, modern habits, nutrient-depleted diets, environmental stressors, and sedentary routines, have created a disconnect between how we live and what the body truly needs to stay resilient. For many, conventional solutions haven't fully addressed these patterns, leaving people still searching for support that feels both effective and sustainable.

That's what *The Medicine-Free, Illness-Free Series* is here to explore.

This series introduces practical, natural options that may help support energy, digestion, sleep, focus, mood, and more, without requiring major lifestyle changes or complicated routines.

It doesn't reject conventional medicine. It expands your toolkit. While modern treatments often focus on managing symptoms in the short term, natural health practices are designed to work more gradually, supporting the body's natural rhythms over time. Many people are rediscovering how ancient practices and modern science can work together, not in opposition, to create a more balanced, resilient life.

The Medicine-Free, Illness-Free Series is built on two foundational pillars:

Science-Informed Solution Benefits: exploring what modern research says about the potential benefits associated with each supplement or therapy

Customer-Reported Solution Benefits: drawn from thousands of real-world user feedback to highlight what people most often experience in practice, including common benefit themes, typical use case patterns, and key user insights.

By combining scientific research with traditional use and real-world user feedback, each volume empowers you to make informed decisions, grounded in both evidence and everyday reality.

Each book in the series focuses on one category of natural therapies. Whether you're exploring Herbal Therapy, Mushroom Therapy, Amino Acid support, Animal Organ Supplements, Grounding, the HOPED Protocol, or detoxification, the goal is the same: to offer trusted solutions that fit easily into your life, simply, naturally, and sustainably.

You don't need to overhaul your lifestyle or commit to an elaborate health plan. You can begin right where you are. Even one small step, a single herb, nutrient, or daily practice, can help you create a rhythm of care that supports your body more naturally over time.

Preface

While no approach guarantees results, many people have found these natural strategies helpful in supporting comfort, energy, focus, and overall vitality. This series was created to help you explore those tools with clarity and confidence, without pressure or complexity.

This volume focuses on Amino Acid Therapy, offering practical insight into key amino acids that support mood, focus, energy, and metabolic health. You'll learn about each amino acid through both research and real-world perspectives, so you can decide what feels right for your journey.

Thank you for beginning this exploration.

Let's move forward, one natural step at a time.

The Medicine-Free, Illness-Free Series

The Medicine-Free, Illness-Free Series is your go-to resource for practical, research-informed natural strategies that are easy to apply. Each volume focuses on a single modality or system—herbs, mushrooms, organ supplements, amino acids, grounding, detox, and more—offering clear guidance to help you choose what works best for you.

Together, the 10 books provide a comprehensive yet flexible wellness framework that supports both daily health maintenance and targeted support. Here's a brief overview of what you'll find in each book:

The Medicine-Free, Illness-Free Series: Why Natural Health Is the Future

Explore why millions of people are turning to nature-aligned strategies to support their wellness. This foundational volume introduces the core science and philosophy behind natural approaches to health, and how they may support your sense of balance, vitality, and overall well-being.

The Medicine-Free, Illness-Free Series: Herbal Therapy

Learn how the world's most time-tested plants may support digestion, energy, relaxation, immune strength, and more. Discover practical ways to include them in your routine and how to choose herbs that match your personal needs and constitution.

The Medicine-Free, Illness-Free Series: Mushroom Therapy

Discover the unique compounds found in medicinal mushrooms that may support immunity, cognitive function, and stress resilience. This book explains how to use mushrooms such as Reishi, Lion's Mane, and Cordyceps in a daily supplement.

The Medicine-Free, Illness-Free Series: Animal Organ Therapy

Explore how nutrient-dense organ supplements, like liver, heart, and kidney, may provide highly bioavailable vitamins, minerals, and peptides. Learn how these traditional foods may support foundational wellness in areas like energy, endurance, and metabolic balance.

The Medicine-Free, Illness-Free Series: Amino Acid Therapy

Uncover the role of amino acids, the building blocks of life, in supporting mood, focus, muscle strength, and nervous system health. This volume shows how targeted amino acid support may help restore clarity, resilience, and emotional well-being.

The Medicine-Free, Illness-Free Series: HOPED Protocol

Learn the five foundational nutrient categories—High Fiber, Omega-3s & Antioxidants, Probiotics, Enzymes, and Vitamin D—and how to implement them as a core wellness strategy. HOPED is simple, actionable, and designed for everyday consistency.

The Medicine-Free, Illness-Free Series: Detoxification Therapy

Discover a gentle, nature-based approach to support your body's natural detoxification processes, promote balance, and encourage overall vitality using simple, practical techniques.

The Medicine-Free, Illness-Free Series: Grounding Therapy

Explore the science and practice of grounding (earthing), the natural process of reconnecting with the Earth's electrical field. Learn how this subtle practice may help support nervous system regulation, sleep quality, and emotional balance.

The Medicine-Free, Illness-Free Series: Diet, Lifestyle and Emotional Well-being

While drastic changes are not required, this volume introduces simple habits that promote long-term balance, covering food, movement, sleep, and emotional self-regulation in a way that aligns with the rest of your natural health plan.

The Medicine-Free, Illness-Free Series: Integrative Therapies for Everyday Health

This final volume brings together insights from the entire series, offering user-reported tools to help support everyday wellness goals, such as energy, digestion, sleep, immunity, and emotional resilience. It serves as a cross-reference for applying the therapies in complementary ways, helping you navigate your health journey with clarity and confidence.

Meet Dr. Forest Yin, DAOM, L.Ac.

Professionally known as Forest Yin, my official name is Jie Yin, while also known as 尹明杰 in the Chinese speaking communities.

For most of my professional life, I was known as a high-tech executive, problem-solver, and innovator in information security and technologies. In leadership roles at Oracle, Schwab, and Wells Fargo, I developed and managed advanced security solutions, ensuring stability, efficiency, and high performance in a fast-paced, high-stakes environment.

But after work, I was deeply immersed in another world, the science of natural health.

My journey into Traditional Chinese Medicine (TCM) began in college, when I first studied the *Huang Di Nei Jing (Yellow Emperor's Classic of Internal Medicine)* alongside my Physics degree. While excelling in my tech career, I continued to research, experiment, and apply natural healing principles, seeking ways to optimize health, energy, and resilience, not just for myself, but for those around me.

Recognizing the profound impact of natural medicine on long-term health and performance, I pursued formal training, becoming a Licensed Acupuncturist (L.Ac.) in 2018 and earning my Doctorate in Acupuncture and Oriental Medicine (DAOM) in 2019. Since then, I have supported individuals around the world in improving their vitality, resilience, and sense of well-being through natural methods. This led me to found Ashi Healing and Acupuncture Inc. and become a Professor and Doctoral Advisor at the University of East-West Medicine, where I mentor future practitioners in the art of TCM.

Applying Systems Thinking to Health & Healing

In high-tech, solving problems requires understanding systems, identifying vulnerabilities, and optimizing performance. I apply the same mindset to health. Instead of treating symptoms, I look at the root cause, like debugging a system. Instead of temporary fixes, I focus on long-term balance and resilience, like designing sustainable architecture. Instead of pharmaceutical dependency, I seek efficient, natural approaches that support function and balance gently, without the common side effects associated with conventional options, like optimizing system performance.

While many of my colleagues in the tech and finance industries thrived in their careers, I also saw the toll of chronic stress, burnout, autoimmune conditions, and lifestyle-related illnesses. Like many professionals, they pushed their limits, until their bodies pushed back. This is where natural approaches can make a difference.

A Philosophy Rooted in Balance & Natural Healing

At Ashi Healing, my approach complements conventional care by focusing on identifying underlying imbalances and supporting the body's natural self-regulation through Traditional Chinese Medicine and holistic strategies.

The name "Ashi (阿是)" comes from a fundamental concept in Chinese medicine, that moment of realization when healing feels real. In Chinese, "Ashi" means "Ahh, Yes!", the instant when your body recognizes exactly what it needs. This guiding philosophy shapes everything I do, from acupuncture to natural health solutions.

Through the precise use of Chinese Herbal Medicine and modern whole-food-based natural supplements like herbs and mushrooms, I have helped individuals support their energy and balance naturally, using simple, sustainable tools that complement or reduce the need for pharmaceutical interventions when appropriate.

My mission is simple: to help people pursue wellness and resilience, naturally and sustainably.

Integrating Ancient Wisdom with Modern Innovation

Chinese Herbal Medicine has been refined for thousands of years. But today, we can take it further, combining ancient wisdom with modern research and a strategic, data-driven approach to health optimization.

At Ashi Healing, I personalize each protocol based on the individual's needs, whether it's boosting energy, reducing stress, improving cognitive function, or addressing chronic health concerns. Many of the people I work with are busy professionals seeking practical, time-efficient strategies to support their health without disrupting their demanding schedules.

Looking for More Information and Support

To learn more about my personalized approach to Chinese Herbal Therapy and whole-food-based supplements, visit AshiHealing.com. You'll find additional resources and simple ways to take the next step in your healing journey, whenever you're ready.

And remember, this book is just one part of *The Medicine-Free, Illness-Free Series*. Each volume explores a different pillar of natural healing, from herbs and mushrooms to amino acids, detoxification, and grounding, offering you a complete path to support your balance and well-being through nature-based strategies.

A Science-Backed, Real-World Tested Method

In *The Medicine-Free, Illness-Free Series*, we introduce a unique, structured method for exploring natural supplements, one that blends scientific insight with real-world observations. Rather than relying solely on clinical studies or anecdotal reports, we combine both perspectives to give you a well-rounded, user-friendly understanding of each natural solution.

This balanced approach helps answer the most important questions: What does science suggest about this supplement's potential? What are people actually experiencing when they use it? Which health goals do people turn to it for most often?

Our method reflects a commitment to transparency, education, and practicality, so you can explore these natural options with clarity and confidence.

Our Four-Part Analysis Method

1. Science-Informed Solution Benefits

We begin by reviewing peer-reviewed studies, traditional usage patterns, and emerging scientific literature to understand the possible mechanisms and effects of each supplement. This provides a foundation of what is known, hypothesized, or being actively researched, offering a science-informed perspective to guide your exploration.

2. Customer-Reported Solution Benefits

We analyze large sets of customer reviews from publicly available platforms to understand how these supplements are being used in daily life. This includes what benefits people say they notice most often and how they describe their experiences.

Our focus is on patterns of what users commonly report, rather than isolated stories. This real-world layer helps connect the theory to practical, everyday outcomes.

3. Use Case Patterns & Feedback Insights

Within the customer-reported section, we highlight:

Use Case Patterns Observed – What kinds of goals or wellness concerns people most commonly use each supplement for.

Feedback Insights – How users describe the impact in their own words, including sentiment, language tone, and satisfaction cues.

Most Reported Benefits – A percentage-based summary showing which benefits are mentioned most often in reviews.

This structured summary lets you see what real people are using the supplement for, and how frequently those benefits are reported.

4. No Brand Promotion—Just Trusted Guidance

This series does not promote specific products or brands. Instead, we offer education and a decision-making framework. For those looking for high-quality sources, recommended supplement types and vetted options are available at AshiHealing.com.

Why This Method Matters

In today's crowded supplement market, it can be hard to separate hype from helpful information. That's why we created this approach, to empower you with insights drawn from scientific research, real-world usage patterns and satisfaction trends, and clear summaries that help you compare options and set expectations

You won't find exaggerated claims or one-size-fits-all solutions here. Instead, you'll find a practical, transparent method that reflects how real people are exploring natural wellness, with science as a guide and personal experience as a reference.

Whether you're considering herbs, mushrooms, amino acids, or other supplements, this method gives you a safe and structured way to learn how others are using these tools, and how they might fit into your own wellness journey.

A Personal Commitment from Dr. Forest Yin

Every approach, strategy, and supplement featured in *The Medicine-Free, Illness-Free Series* has been personally explored. Before sharing any recommendations with clients or readers, I take the time to experience it myself, observing how it affects energy, mood, sleep, digestion, and focus.

This hands-on approach allows me to understand each therapy not just through science, or just through other people's experiences. It adds a personal layer of insight to the research and user-reported feedback that shape this series.

My goal is simple: to help you find natural, sustainable solutions that feel doable, helpful, and aligned with how lasting wellness begins, by reconnecting with your body's own rhythms and innate intelligence

Harness the Potential of Amino Acid Therapy

Amino acid therapy is increasingly recognized as a natural, science-informed approach to supporting overall health and well-being. Known as the "building blocks of life," amino acids form the foundation of proteins and are involved in nearly every physiological process in the body. From supporting muscle function and energy production to influencing mental focus and emotional resilience, amino acids are essential to maintaining internal balance.

Modern life, with its fast pace, chronic stress, and nutritional gaps, can contribute to imbalances or deficiencies in key amino acids. Targeted amino acid supplementation may help restore that balance and provide nutritional support in areas such as vitality, cognitive performance, and physical recovery. For those dealing with low energy, mental fatigue, or physical strain, amino acid therapy offers a proactive way to reinforce the body's natural systems.

Rather than focusing on short-term fixes, this form of nutritional support is both restorative and preventive. By understanding how specific amino acids contribute to overall health, individuals can take meaningful steps to build strength, focus, and resilience through natural and sustainable means.

A Brief History of Amino Acid Therapy

While amino acid therapy may seem like a modern innovation, its foundation dates back to the early 19th century with the discovery of amino acids themselves. Initially explored for their role in protein synthesis, these vital compounds gradually gained recognition for their broader significance in human health.

By the 20th century, researchers had begun to identify the impact of amino acid imbalances and deficiencies on various aspects of physical and mental function. In clinical settings, amino acid-based nutritional formulas were introduced to support recovery from surgery, malnutrition, or intense physical stress.

In the decades that followed, particularly during the 1960s and 1970s, scientific interest expanded to include the potential role of amino acids in supporting mood, energy, and performance. This growing body of research gave rise to what is now referred to as amino acid therapy: the intentional use of specific amino acids to support physiological processes and promote overall well-being.

Today, amino acid therapy is part of many holistic and integrative wellness strategies. Whether used by athletes to support physical performance or by individuals seeking natural ways to feel better, amino acids provide a personalized and flexible approach to self-care that aligns with modern health goals.

The Role of Amino Acids in Health

Amino acids are essential to virtually every biological function in the human body. As the fundamental components of proteins, they help form the structure of muscles, skin, hair, and internal organs. Yet their influence goes far beyond physical structure. Amino acids also serve as precursors to neurotransmitters, chemical messengers in the brain that play a role in regulating mood, memory, focus, and sleep. Because of this, amino acids are often associated with supporting cognitive and emotional balance.

One of the most widely appreciated aspects of amino acids is their role in maintaining and rebuilding muscle tissue. For individuals who are physically active, recovering from strain, or seeking to maintain strength over time, amino acids, including branched-chain amino acids (BCAAs), may help support muscle recovery, maintenance, and overall physical performance. They are also involved in supporting immune system function by contributing to the production of key proteins that help defend the body.

In terms of metabolism and energy, amino acids help facilitate the breakdown of nutrients for energy, support healthy blood sugar regulation, and assist in the body's natural detoxification processes by participating in liver function. Their involvement in hormone production and regulation further highlights their importance, especially for individuals navigating fluctuations in energy, mood, or reproductive health.

Unlike many generalized approaches to wellness, amino acid therapy allows for targeted support. Each amino acid offers specific contributions to different areas of well-being, which means supplementation can often be tailored to your body's unique needs. Whether you're looking to maintain energy levels, support mental focus, or aid muscle recovery, amino acids can play a valuable role in a personalized health strategy.

The Role of Amino Acids in Healthy Aging

Amino acids are also gaining attention for their potential to support graceful aging. They contribute to the body's production of collagen and elastin, two proteins essential for maintaining skin elasticity and firmness. By supporting these structural proteins, amino acids may help promote a more youthful appearance over time.

Some amino acids also have antioxidant properties, which means they may help the body manage oxidative stress and reduce the impact of free radicals, unstable molecules that are associated with age-related cellular changes. Additionally, amino acids are involved in preserving lean muscle mass, supporting liver function, and promoting detoxification, all of which are important for maintaining strength, vitality, and overall resilience as we age.

Beyond physical health, amino acids also play roles in supporting cognitive function and mood. This makes them an appealing option for individuals seeking to maintain clarity, focus, and emotional well-being through every stage of life. When incorporated into a thoughtful self-care routine, amino acid therapy may provide a gentle, natural way to promote long-term wellness and vitality.

Essential vs. Non-Essential Amino Acids

Amino acids are the foundational components of proteins and play important roles in nearly every biological process in the body. In this book, they are grouped into two main categories, Essential Amino Acids (EAAs) and Non-Essential Amino Acids (non-EAAs), each with unique contributions to physical performance, mental focus, emotional stability, and overall well-being.

Essential Amino Acids (EAAs) are classified as "essential" because the body cannot produce them on its own. They must be obtained through diet or supplementation. Without adequate intake of all nine EAAs, the body may not efficiently build proteins, support recovery, or maintain optimal cellular function. This book highlights the nine essential amino acids: Lysine, Tryptophan, Methionine, Phenylalanine, Leucine, Isoleucine, Valine, Threonine, and Histidine. While each plays a distinct role in supporting health, their most effective impact is often seen when they are used in combination. Together, they contribute to protein synthesis, cognitive performance, and the maintenance of lean muscle.

Non-Essential Amino Acids may be produced by the body under typical conditions, but that doesn't mean they are always available in sufficient amounts. Factors such as stress, aging, illness, or inadequate nutrition can increase the demand for certain amino acids, making supplementation beneficial in some cases. This book explores several non-essential and conditionally essential amino acids that are valued for their supportive roles in wellness. These include N-Acetyl Cysteine (NAC), Glutathione, Glycine, Tyrosine, Carnitine, Arginine, Serine, L-Theanine, GABA, Taurine, D-Aspartic Acid, and Glutamine. Each contributes to functions such as antioxidant support, energy metabolism, neurotransmitter activity, and cellular protection.

By understanding the complementary roles of both essential and non-essential amino acids, readers can better navigate how targeted supplementation may fit into a broader natural health strategy.

My Journey with Amino Acid Therapy

As a practitioner of Traditional Chinese Medicine, I've always been passionate about exploring the full spectrum of natural healing approaches. Over the years, I've studied a wide range of therapies, from time-tested herbal remedies to the latest in integrative health strategies. Among the many tools I've encountered, one that stood out for its simplicity and effectiveness was amino acid therapy.

My interest began when a longtime client, an avid distance runner, shared his experience using essential amino acids to support his recovery and performance. After months of struggling to bounce back from a lingering injury, he noticed a marked improvement after incorporating amino acids into his routine. His story piqued my curiosity and led me to explore the research and applications of these foundational nutrients.

Wanting to understand their effects more personally, I began experimenting with amino acids in my own life. The results were noticeable. I felt more physically resilient during exercise, recovered more smoothly after exertion, and even noticed improvements in sleep quality and overall mood. These changes, while subtle at first, became more consistent over time and inspired me to look deeper into how amino acids work within the body.

Since then, I've gradually integrated amino acid protocols into my practice as part of a broader natural health strategy. While every individual's needs are unique, I've found that amino acids offer a flexible and accessible way to support strength, focus, and recovery. They've become an important part of my toolkit for promoting balance and well-being, both in my own life and in the lives of those I work with.

What to Expect in This Book

This book uses a science-informed, real-world-tested approach to explore the potential of amino acid therapy. Each amino acid is examined through a structured lens designed to help you make informed and confident decisions about incorporating amino acids into your wellness routine.

Here's what you'll find in each amino acid profile:

Science-Informed Solution Benefits

This section introduces the physiological role of each amino acid and highlights areas of ongoing research. You'll learn how each amino acid contributes to functions such as neurotransmitter production, muscle recovery, energy metabolism, or hormonal balance. These insights are based on peer-reviewed studies, established biochemistry, and the known mechanisms by which amino acids support overall well-being. This section focuses on potential areas of support, not on treatment or disease outcomes.

Customer-Reported Solution Benefits

To provide a clearer view of how people experience amino acids in everyday life, we've analyzed patterns in real-world feedback.

Use Case Patterns Observed: This section highlights the most common reasons people choose a specific amino acid. It reflects user motivations such as supporting mental clarity, stress resilience, recovery, or energy.

Feedback Insights: This narrative summary shares how users describe their experiences, capturing both functional and emotional responses. It reveals how people report feeling after using each amino acid, based on the language and tone seen across verified reviews.

Most Reported Benefits from Review Analysis: This table and accompanying summary highlight the top benefits mentioned in real-world feedback, based on frequency of mention. It gives you a quick overview of what users most often notice.

Reference Guide to Everyday Health Goals

At the end of the book, you'll find a cross-reference section that links commonly mentioned health goals, such as stress support, mood balance, energy, or focus, with the amino acids most frequently associated with those outcomes. This guide is based on both science-informed understanding and user feedback trends. It is intended for educational purposes and not as a substitute for professional medical advice.

By combining scientific insight with real-world observations, this book offers a balanced and practical guide to amino acid therapy. Whether you're looking to support muscle recovery, enhance focus, or maintain emotional well-being, you'll find tools in these pages to help you move forward naturally and effectively.

Lysine

Lysine is an essential amino acid that plays a vital role in overall health, including skin integrity, immune function, and tissue support. It contributes to the production of collagen, a key structural protein in the skin, which helps maintain a firm, smooth appearance. Lysine also supports the body's natural defenses and plays a role in bone health and muscle recovery.

Many people incorporate lysine into their wellness routines as part of a proactive approach to maintaining clear skin, physical resilience, and overall vitality. Whether you're looking to support your skin, strengthen your body, or simply enhance your self-care regimen, lysine offers foundational support for health from the inside out.

Science-Informed Lysine Benefits

Lysine is an essential amino acid that contributes to a wide range of physiological functions. It plays a critical role in supporting skin structure, immune system function, bone strength, and nutrient absorption. Because the body cannot produce lysine on its own, it must be obtained through diet or supplementation. Below are key areas where lysine has been studied and recognized for its biological significance.

Support for Skin Structure and Appearance

Lysine is directly involved in the production of collagen, a structural protein responsible for maintaining skin elasticity and firmness. Adequate lysine intake supports the body's natural ability to maintain skin integrity, which may contribute to a smoother, more even appearance over time. Some research also suggests that lysine plays a role in tissue repair, helping the body maintain a healthy response to minor skin damage and promoting efficient recovery. Because of its contribution to collagen formation and cell regeneration, lysine is often included in wellness routines aimed at supporting skin resilience and maintaining a youthful look.

Immune Function and Viral Defense

Lysine has been widely studied for its role in supporting immune function. It is believed to influence the body's response to stress and immune challenges by supporting the production of immune-related proteins and enzymes. Some research also suggests that lysine may help regulate the activity of certain viruses by competing with other amino acids that viruses rely on to replicate. While not a treatment, lysine's involvement in these processes makes it a useful addition to immune-support protocols.

Calcium Absorption and Bone Health

Lysine helps the body absorb and retain calcium, a mineral essential for maintaining healthy bones and teeth. By supporting calcium transport and utilization, lysine plays a supportive role in skeletal strength and long-term bone maintenance. In addition, lysine is involved in collagen cross-linking, which contributes to the structural integrity of both bone tissue and connective tissue. These properties make lysine a valuable nutrient for those interested in supporting bone density and oral health.

Customer-Reported Lysine Benefits

Lysine has quietly become a go-to supplement for many individuals seeking lasting support for clearer skin, stronger immunity, and fewer disruptions from cold sores or other recurring issues. With thousands of positive reviews and a strong average rating of 4.6 out of 5, users consistently describe it as a "life-changing" addition to their wellness routine. Whether discovered in a moment of frustration or recommended by a trusted source, lysine is often described not just as helpful, but as something that made people feel like themselves again. Its impact is rarely dramatic overnight, but for many, the changes are surprisingly fast and deeply felt, especially when other options have failed. Those who stick with it often speak of restored confidence, fewer flare-ups, and a new sense of control over their skin and health.

Use Case Patterns Observed

Many users first turn to lysine after long-standing struggles with skin-related concerns, especially cold sores, canker sores, or recurring breakouts that seem to defy every other approach. Some found it through late-night research, while others were encouraged by a friend, a YouTube video, or even a suggestion from their doctor. For individuals dealing with hormonal acne or outbreaks triggered by stress, lysine often becomes a daily ritual and a form of maintenance they trust. Cold sore sufferers frequently report using lysine both as a preventative measure and for faster recovery, often taking higher doses at the first sign of a tingle or flare-up.

Others begin using lysine for its broader benefits, such as improved healing, more even skin tone, and immune support during times of stress or seasonal illness. There are also a number of reviewers who discovered its usefulness through more complex journeys, including shingles flare-ups, mouth sensitivities, or nutrient absorption challenges related to gut health. Across these use cases, the pattern is consistent: lysine isn't just a reactive supplement for acute problems, but something people incorporate into daily routines to maintain balance, confidence, and resilience.

Feedback Insights

What stands out most in the reviews is the deep emotional relief users describe, especially from those who had tried many solutions with little success. One user called lysine "a God-send" after eight years of struggling with acne on back and neck at age 74, while another said they were "over the moon excited" after finally seeing their hormonal acne clear up when nothing else had worked. Many cold sore sufferers described years of feeling embarrassed or defeated by recurring outbreaks, only to find that lysine helped reduce both their frequency and intensity. They speak of fewer flare-ups, faster healing, and a new sense of freedom in their social and professional lives.

Several reviewers emphasized how quickly they noticed changes, using phrases like "life-changing," "improved overnight," or "crazy how well it works." Some shared that they were skeptical at first but deeply moved when their skin improved or their outbreaks subsided. For many, lysine brought a feeling of control after years of unpredictability. Others appreciated unexpected benefits, such as brighter skin tone, less stress, or improved wound healing.

The overwhelming sentiment is clear: for those who have struggled with skin sensitivity, immune concerns, or recurring flare-ups, lysine often feels like a quiet but powerful shift, something simple that finally made a real difference.

Most Reported Benefits from Review Analysis

To better understand what users are actually experiencing, we conducted a deep analysis of thousands of verified customer reviews, focusing on the benefits most frequently mentioned by satisfied users. The table below reflects the distribution of reported benefits across thousands of positive experiences with lysine. While individual results may vary, a higher percentage suggests a more consistent pattern of benefit shared by others.

For example, 56 percent of reviewers specifically mentioned a noticeable reduction in cold sore frequency and severity, suggesting that if you are using lysine for this purpose, there is a strong likelihood you may experience a similar outcome. Likewise, improvements in skin clarity and immune support were consistently highlighted, painting a picture of a supplement that supports both resilience and appearance in everyday life.

Below is a summary table of lysine's top benefits as reported by customers:

Benefit	%	Explanation
Cold Sore Support	56%	Most users report fewer outbreaks, faster healing, and greater overall control.
Skin Health & Clarity	22%	Many reviewers mention reduced acne, clearer complexion, and fewer irritations.
Immune Function	14%	A consistent number of users say they feel less run down or get sick less often.
Stress and Mood	8%	A smaller group reports improved emotional balance and reduced daily tension.

How to Use This Guide

If you are considering lysine for a specific wellness goal such as cold sore management, clearer skin, or general immune support, these insights offer a helpful reference. The percentages reflect how often each benefit is mentioned by real users, not a guarantee of individual results. However, they do reveal which outcomes are most frequently noticed and appreciated in real-world use.

Keep in mind that many users report experiencing more than one benefit at a time, especially with consistent daily use. Whether you are just beginning your wellness journey or looking to fine-tune your routine, lysine's strong track record makes it a well-regarded option for targeted support.

Tryptophan

Tryptophan is an essential amino acid best known for its role in supporting emotional balance, restful sleep, and overall vitality. As a fundamental building block of protein, tryptophan contributes to muscle maintenance and recovery, but its influence reaches far beyond the musculoskeletal system. It plays a critical role in the production of key neurotransmitters and hormones that help regulate mood, manage stress, and promote deep, restorative sleep. Because the body cannot produce tryptophan on its own, it must be obtained through diet or supplementation.

For those seeking to support a calm mind, more consistent sleep patterns, or clearer skin, tryptophan is often included as part of a daily wellness routine. It is valued not only for what it helps the body produce, such as serotonin and melatonin, but also for the way it contributes to a more grounded, resilient state of well-being over time.

Science-Informed Tryptophan Benefits

Tryptophan has been widely studied for its role in regulating neurotransmitter activity, sleep cycles, and immune function. Its physiological impact is rooted in its conversion into serotonin and melatonin, both of which are crucial to emotional and physical balance.

Mood and Emotional Well-Being

Tryptophan is a necessary precursor for the synthesis of serotonin, a neurotransmitter involved in regulating mood, appetite, and emotional processing. Low serotonin levels are associated with emotional imbalances, while adequate levels are linked to a greater sense of calm and well-being. Supplementing with tryptophan may help support a more stable emotional baseline and promote positive outlook, especially during periods of stress or change. Some research also suggests it plays a role in maintaining cognitive focus, making it a popular option for those seeking to support both emotional clarity and mental performance.

Sleep Support

As a precursor to melatonin, the hormone that governs the body's natural sleep-wake rhythm, tryptophan is closely connected to sleep quality. Studies have shown that increased tryptophan intake may help reduce the time it takes to fall asleep, improve sleep continuity, and enhance overall restfulness. This makes tryptophan a popular choice for those experiencing occasional sleep disruptions or wanting to maintain more consistent rest patterns. Its gentle support for sleep architecture makes it a well-tolerated option for natural nighttime support.

Skin Health and Recovery

Tryptophan contributes to the body's production of collagen, the structural protein responsible for skin firmness and elasticity. This link to collagen synthesis makes tryptophan an indirect supporter of skin resilience and renewal. In addition, it has been studied for its antioxidant and anti-inflammatory properties, which may play a role in soothing skin sensitivity and supporting tissue repair. Some users incorporate it into their routines to help maintain a more even complexion or to support overall skin wellness as part of an anti-aging approach.

Additional Areas of Support

Beyond its better-known benefits, tryptophan has been explored for its role in supporting relaxation during occasional episodes of heightened stress or nervous tension. It may also influence muscle comfort by supporting neurotransmitter balance, which in turn may affect how muscles respond to overexertion. Additionally, serotonin plays a role in immune system communication, and by contributing to serotonin production, tryptophan may help support the body's natural defenses.

Customer-Reported L-Tryptophan Benefits

L-Tryptophan has earned a strong reputation among those seeking deeper, more restful sleep, greater emotional balance, and a gentler alternative to conventional approaches for anxiety or mood support. With thousands of positive reviews and a solid average rating of 4.5 out of 5 stars, many users describe it as a transformative part of their wellness routines. While the reasons for trying L-Tryptophan vary, from chronic insomnia to the desire for more natural emotional support, what unites most stories is a deep sense of relief and renewed stability. For many, it becomes the first supplement they've tried that truly makes a noticeable difference, often after years of frustration with other options.

Use Case Patterns Observed

L-Tryptophan is most commonly discovered by individuals navigating long-standing issues with sleep, mood regulation, or chronic stress. Many reviewers mentioned trying prescription medications in the past, often with side effects or diminishing returns, before seeking out a more natural alternative. Others turn to L-Tryptophan after learning it is a precursor to serotonin and melatonin, which sparked curiosity about its potential for both sleep quality and emotional well-being.

Among the most common patterns, users report taking L-Tryptophan in the evening to ease into sleep, often combining it with magnesium, GABA, or theanine. Those with anxiety often take smaller doses during the day to support calm and focus. Several individuals who had previously struggled with early morning waking, restless nights, or racing thoughts describe L-Tryptophan as the turning point in restoring restful sleep. A significant number of reviewers also use it alongside other amino acids, like L-Tyrosine, as part of a balanced mood-support regimen. For some, its benefits emerge gradually; for others, the change is felt within days.

Feedback Insights

Reviewers frequently use words like *calm*, *centered*, *balanced*, and *relieved* to describe their experiences. Many share that they "finally sleep through the night" or wake up "refreshed for the first time in years." Several note a striking difference in how they feel both emotionally and physically, explaining that they no longer dread bedtime or fear the exhaustion that used to follow a poor night's sleep.

Others reflect on how much their anxiety and irritability diminished over time, with one user saying they feel "comfortable in their own skin again." Another described it as a "game-changer," crediting L-Tryptophan with helping them reclaim a sense of normalcy without dependency or grogginess. There is also a recurring theme of gratitude for a product that supports emotional resilience without the side effects commonly associated with pharmaceutical options.

What stands out most is the emotional depth of the testimonials. Users often write not just about improved sleep or mood, but about the ripple effect it has had on their relationships, confidence, and sense of control. For some, L-Tryptophan became the first supplement that made them feel truly hopeful again.

Most Reported Benefits from Review Analysis

To better understand how L-Tryptophan is experienced in everyday use, we analyzed thousands of verified customer reviews and identified the benefits most frequently reported by satisfied users. The table below reflects the distribution of positive outcomes shared across a large pool of feedback. While individual results can vary, a higher percentage suggests a more consistent benefit observed by others with similar goals.

For example, 55 percent of reviewers highlighted improved sleep quality, suggesting that if restful sleep is a priority, L-Tryptophan may be particularly helpful. Many users also mentioned a greater sense of calm, reduced nervous tension, and better mood balance after consistent use.

Below is a summary table of L-Tryptophan's top benefits as reported by customers:

Benefit	%	Explanation
Sleep Support	55%	Most users describe falling asleep faster, staying asleep longer, and waking up feeling more rested.
Mood Improvement	19%	Many note a noticeable uplift in daily outlook and emotional resilience, often describing a more even, steady mood.
Anxiety and Stress	18%	A significant portion of users mention feeling calmer and more relaxed, especially during times of stress or overstimulation.
Emotional Low Points	7%	Some users report feeling more emotionally balanced and supported during difficult or low-energy periods.

How to Use This Guide

If you are considering L-Tryptophan to support restful sleep, a calmer mindset, or improved emotional well-being, this data offers a helpful starting point. The percentages reflect how often each benefit was mentioned, not a guarantee of results. However, they do offer real-world insight into how others have used this supplement to support their goals.

Many users report experiencing more than one benefit, especially with consistent daily use over several weeks. Whether you are exploring natural sleep support, emotional clarity, or simply a more relaxed state of being, L-Tryptophan's steady track record makes it one of the most trusted amino acid supplements available today.

Methionine

Methionine is an essential amino acid that supports a wide range of biological functions, making it a valuable addition to any wellness routine. As a key nutrient that the body cannot produce on its own, methionine must be obtained through diet or supplementation. It plays a central role in detoxification, antioxidant activity, protein synthesis, and cellular health. Its contributions to liver support, skin and hair maintenance, and metabolic function make it particularly noteworthy for those seeking to promote internal balance and external vitality.

Whether your goal is to maintain liver function, protect against oxidative stress, or support skin and hair health, Methionine offers versatile support that can help maintain your body's natural resilience and performance.

Science-Informed Methionine Benefits

Methionine is best known for its contributions to detoxification, antioxidant defense, and protein metabolism. Its biochemical roles are fundamental to maintaining tissue integrity, supporting cellular processes, and enhancing overall vitality.

Detoxification and Liver Support

Methionine is a key precursor to glutathione, a vital compound involved in the body's natural detoxification system. Glutathione helps neutralize reactive molecules and supports the breakdown and removal of metabolic byproducts and environmental toxins. By helping to sustain healthy glutathione levels, methionine plays an important role in promoting liver efficiency and resilience.

Additionally, it assists in the transport and metabolism of fats, helping to prevent excess fat from accumulating in the liver. These properties make methionine an important nutrient for maintaining liver health under normal physiological conditions.

Antioxidant Activity and Cellular Defense

Through its involvement in glutathione synthesis, methionine supports the body's natural antioxidant systems. This function helps protect tissues from oxidative stress, a process associated with cellular damage and accelerated aging. Methionine's role in neutralizing free radicals also contributes to the maintenance of long-term cellular integrity. In this way, it may help support the body's defenses against environmental stressors and contribute to a sense of energy and well-being over time.

Skin, Hair, and Nail Support

Methionine plays a role in the synthesis of collagen and keratin, two structural proteins critical for maintaining the strength and elasticity of skin, hair, and nails. By supporting protein formation and tissue regeneration, methionine contributes to a healthy complexion, strong nails, and resilient hair. Some individuals include methionine in their self-care routines to promote smoother skin texture, improve hair shine, and reduce the appearance of damage or brittleness.

Muscle Health and Protein Metabolism

As a building block of proteins, methionine is essential for tissue repair and muscle maintenance. It plays a foundational role in protein synthesis, helping to preserve lean muscle mass and support recovery following physical activity. For athletes or those with active lifestyles, methionine may support overall physical performance by contributing to energy production pathways and muscle resilience.

Methylation and Cardiovascular Function

Methionine is involved in the body's methylation cycle, a process that supports DNA function, neurotransmitter balance, and overall metabolic health. It helps regulate homocysteine levels by contributing to the conversion of homocysteine back into methionine through vitamin-dependent pathways. Maintaining balanced homocysteine levels is one way to support cardiovascular health, making methionine a key player in nutritional strategies for heart and circulatory wellness.

Customer-Reported Methionine Benefits

Unlike Lysine or L-Tryptophan, Methionine is rarely taken alone and is usually found in amino acid complexes or liver support formulas. It plays key roles in detoxification, antioxidant production (glutathione), joint health, and keratin formation for hair and nails. It also supports mood balance via SAMe synthesis but may raise homocysteine levels without enough B6, B12, and Folate. Due to its limited standalone use, customer feedback is scarce. Instead, Methionine is best discussed alongside Cysteine (NAC) and Taurine, which share similar functions and are more widely supplemented.

Phenylalanine

Phenylalanine is an essential amino acid with a wide range of functions that support both physical and mental well-being. As a key component in protein synthesis, it also serves as a precursor to several important brain chemicals that influence mood, focus, and stress response. Additionally, phenylalanine contributes to the production of melanin, the pigment responsible for skin and hair coloration, offering added value for skin health and appearance.

Since the body cannot produce phenylalanine on its own, it must be obtained through diet or supplementation. Its diverse roles in neurotransmitter function, cognitive performance, and skin biology make it a popular option for those seeking to support emotional balance, mental clarity, and a more vibrant appearance, all through natural, science-informed pathways.

Science-Informed Phenylalanine Benefits

Phenylalanine supports a number of key biological processes, ranging from neurotransmitter production to cellular repair and pigmentation. It is widely studied for its role in supporting brain function, mood regulation, and the appearance of skin.

Mood and Emotional Balance

Phenylalanine is a precursor to dopamine, norepinephrine, and epinephrine, neurotransmitters involved in emotional regulation, alertness, and the body's response to stress. These brain chemicals influence how we feel, how we handle pressure, and how motivated we are to take action. By supporting the body's natural ability to produce these compounds, phenylalanine may help promote a sense of calm, uplifted energy, and improved emotional resilience during times of stress or mental fatigue.

Cognitive Function and Focus

Through its influence on neurotransmitter activity, phenylalanine plays a role in supporting memory, focus, and overall cognitive function. It is commonly included in mental performance supplements aimed at improving clarity and attention span. For individuals who experience occasional brain fog or mental sluggishness, phenylalanine may offer a natural way to support sharper thinking and sustained concentration.

Comfort and Physical Resilience

Phenylalanine has been explored for its influence on the body's pain regulation pathways, particularly in relation to natural endorphin activity. While additional research is ongoing, its ability to support healthy nerve signaling and comfort has made it of interest to individuals managing physical discomfort or seeking added support for resilience during daily activities. It is often combined with other amino acids or nutrients as part of a broader strategy for musculoskeletal support.

Skin Pigmentation and Structural Support

Phenylalanine is involved in the synthesis of melanin, which gives skin and hair their natural pigment. This process also plays a role in how the skin responds to sun exposure. In addition, phenylalanine supports protein synthesis, including the production of collagen, a key structural component for skin elasticity and firmness. These combined effects may contribute to a more even skin tone and enhanced skin texture over time.

Cellular Health and Immune Support

As part of its broader role in protein metabolism, phenylalanine contributes to the maintenance of healthy cells throughout the body. It is involved in enzymatic functions and supports normal immune cell activity. By participating in these essential functions, phenylalanine helps the body maintain balance and resilience in the face of everyday challenges.

Customer-Reported Phenylalanine Benefits

L-Phenylalanine has earned the trust of many individuals seeking a natural way to enhance emotional balance, sharpen mental clarity, and maintain a greater sense of energy and motivation. With an overall customer rating of 4.2 out of 5, this essential amino acid has become a go-to choice for those navigating low mood, difficulty focusing, and daily stress. Users describe a noticeable lift in their mindset, greater resilience, and an improved ability to enjoy everyday life without overstimulation or harsh side effects. Unlike fast-acting stimulants or medications, the changes are often described as subtle at first, but deeply impactful over time. For many, phenylalanine offers a pathway to feeling more present, alert, and capable of handling life's demands with clarity and optimism.

Use Case Patterns Observed

L-Phenylalanine is most often used by individuals experiencing emotional fatigue, cognitive fog, or a lack of drive. Many reviewers shared that they turned to this supplement during periods of low motivation, heightened stress, or when transitioning away from prescription antidepressants. It is commonly used first thing in the morning to support mental clarity and set a more balanced tone for the day. Others began using it in combination with related nutrients like Tyrosine, vitamin B6, or GABA for broader emotional support. While some reviewers seek out phenylalanine as a mood enhancer, others take it as part of a cognitive performance stack to help with attention, focus, or productivity, especially during demanding or stressful work hours. In several cases, users reported pairing it with lifestyle changes such as exercise or healthier eating, noting that phenylalanine seemed to enhance their ability to follow through with those positive routines.

Feedback Insights

The emotional language in phenylalanine reviews often centers around a renewed sense of clarity, lightness, and inner steadiness. One night-shift nurse described waking up for the first time in months with the words, "What a beautiful day," despite no external changes in circumstance, just a subtle but meaningful shift in internal state. Others noted that their sense of well-being felt restored, often saying things like, "I feel like myself again," or "This helped me get back to who I was." For individuals dealing with long-term depression or mood instability, the relief described was both practical and personal. They often expressed gratitude that a single capsule could help lift the "emotional fog" that had clouded their thinking or drained their energy.

Many reviewers also mentioned improved focus and sharper mental function, particularly after a few weeks of consistent use. Some reported feeling more capable of completing tasks or handling daily stress without feeling overwhelmed. A number of users mentioned that phenylalanine helped ease emotional reactivity, with one person saying they were "less easily offended" and felt "steadier" throughout the day. Even skeptics, including medical professionals, shared positive shifts in energy and motivation that felt noticeably different from their previous experiences with prescription medications.

For individuals facing long-standing emotional or cognitive challenges, phenylalanine is often described as a gentle but powerful step toward reclaiming balance, productivity, and emotional resilience.

Most Reported Benefits from Review Analysis

To better understand how people experience phenylalanine in real-world use, we analyzed thousands of verified customer reviews. The data below highlights the benefits most frequently mentioned by satisfied users. While results can vary for each individual, the percentages reflect consistent patterns of use and reported impact.

For instance, nearly 47% of reviewers shared that phenylalanine helped improve their overall mood and emotional balance. This trend suggests that if mood support is a primary concern, phenylalanine may be especially worth considering. Similarly, a significant number of users also reported increases in energy and focus, pointing to its broader support for mental performance and motivation.

Below is a summary table of phenylalanine's most commonly reported benefits:

Benefit	%	Explanation
Mood Enhancement	47%	Many users describe a noticeable uplift in mood, greater emotional steadiness, and a return to a more positive mindset. These effects are likely tied to phenylalanine's role in supporting neurotransmitter activity, including dopamine.

Benefit	%	Explanation
Energy Boost	27%	Users often report feeling more energetic and motivated, particularly during morning hours or after periods of fatigue. Phenylalanine's support for dopamine and adrenal function may play a role.
Focus & Mental Clarity	16%	A notable portion of reviews highlight clearer thinking, reduced brain fog, and better attention span. This makes phenylalanine a popular option for those seeking to stay sharp throughout the day.
Appetite Control	9%	Some users observed reduced cravings or a decreased desire for overeating. This may be related to improved mood regulation and metabolic balance.
Pain Relief	1%	A small but meaningful group shared improvements in discomfort, especially related to long-standing conditions. This benefit appears less common but still noteworthy.

How to Use This Guide

If you're exploring phenylalanine for a specific goal such as improving mood, boosting energy, or supporting focus, these review-based insights can offer helpful direction. The percentages represent how often users mentioned each benefit in positive reviews, not guaranteed outcomes. However, they do reflect what phenylalanine is most commonly appreciated for.

It's also important to remember that benefits are often cumulative. Many users report greater effects after several weeks of consistent use, and some experience multiple benefits at the same time. Whether you're managing daily stress, seeking a natural motivation boost, or simply aiming to feel more balanced, phenylalanine's wide-ranging support makes it a valued option for many.

Leucine

Leucine is a branched-chain essential amino acid (BCAA) that plays a critical role in supporting muscle integrity, metabolic function, and overall vitality. As one of the three BCAAs, alongside isoleucine and valine, leucine is particularly notable for its ability to stimulate protein synthesis and aid in muscle tissue recovery. While it is widely recognized among athletes and active individuals, its benefits extend far beyond the gym. Leucine is essential for maintaining healthy body composition, preserving muscle mass during aging or illness, and supporting stable energy levels. Whether you are aiming to build strength, recover from physical exertion, or maintain your wellness during periods of stress or inactivity, leucine provides powerful support for both physical and metabolic health.

Science-Informed Leucine Benefits

Muscle Growth and Repair

Leucine plays a central role in activating the mTOR signaling pathway, which directly stimulates muscle protein synthesis. This makes leucine particularly effective in promoting the growth and repair of muscle tissue, especially after resistance training or physical exertion. It also helps prevent muscle breakdown by providing essential building blocks for recovery, which is beneficial for individuals experiencing muscle loss due to aging, immobilization, or restricted caloric intake. Maintaining adequate leucine levels is especially important for those undergoing rehabilitation or aiming to preserve lean body mass during weight loss. Leucine may support conditions such as age-related sarcopenia, recovery after surgery or injury, and muscle atrophy.

Metabolic Health

Leucine contributes to metabolic balance by supporting glucose metabolism and improving insulin sensitivity. By enhancing the body's ability to process glucose, leucine plays a role in stabilizing blood sugar levels and supporting overall energy efficiency. In addition, leucine promotes lean muscle development, which helps raise the body's resting metabolic rate. This contributes to more effective calorie utilization and supports long-term weight management. These metabolic effects make leucine a valuable nutrient for individuals managing insulin resistance, metabolic syndrome, or obesity-related challenges.

Energy Production

During prolonged physical activity, fasting, or energy-restricted conditions, leucine can serve as an alternative energy source for the body. It is broken down into compounds that enter the energy cycle, helping to fuel muscle function and delay the onset of fatigue. This makes leucine an important tool for supporting endurance, reducing exercise-related tiredness, and maintaining stamina throughout the day. It is particularly useful for individuals who experience chronic low energy or who engage in sustained physical exertion. Leucine may be supportive in situations involving chronic fatigue, strenuous exercise, or general physical depletion.

Brain Function

While leucine is best known for its physical benefits, it also supports mental performance by participating in the synthesis of neurotransmitters, including glutamate and GABA. These neurotransmitters play vital roles in memory, focus, and stress resilience. By contributing to balanced brain chemistry, leucine helps support cognitive clarity, attention, and mental stamina. It may be particularly beneficial for individuals experiencing cognitive fatigue, brain fog, or attention-related concerns. Leucine's support for neurological function highlights its broader role in whole-body health.

Immune Support

Leucine also plays a role in immune health by supporting the growth and function of immune cells, including lymphocytes. This is particularly important during periods of physical stress, illness, or recovery when the body requires additional resources for repair and defense. By supporting protein synthesis at the cellular level, leucine contributes to a more resilient immune response and helps maintain the body's ability to respond effectively to infections. It may be useful during times of increased immune demand, such as after illness, surgery, or during periods of high physical stress.

Customer-Reported BCAA Benefits

L-Leucine, Isoleucine, and Valine are primarily used together as Branched-Chain Amino Acids (BCAAs) rather than as standalone supplements. While each has distinct functions—Leucine triggers muscle protein synthesis, Isoleucine supports energy regulation, and Valine enhances endurance—they work synergistically and are almost always taken in a 2:1:1 or 3:1:1 ratio for optimal performance. Since most customer reviews focus on BCAA blends, analyzing them separately would provide limited insights. Instead, evaluating BCAAs as a whole gives a more accurate, customer-validated picture of their real-world benefits in muscle recovery, energy, and athletic performance.

Use Case Patterns Observed

Branched-Chain Amino Acids (BCAAs), a blend of leucine, isoleucine, and valine, are frequently used by individuals engaging in strength training, endurance sports, and high-intensity fitness programs. Most users turn to BCAAs for one or more of the following goals: reducing post-exercise soreness, improving workout performance, accelerating recovery, or maintaining muscle mass during caloric restriction or aging. Some reviewers mentioned using BCAAs during fasted workouts to prevent muscle breakdown, while others took them alongside protein powders or within custom pre- or post-workout stacks. Users span a broad range, including CrossFit participants, long-distance cyclists, vegetarians seeking better muscle support, and older adults focused on recovery and stamina.

Although many reviewers combine BCAAs with other ingredients such as creatine, glutamine, or beta-alanine, their feedback consistently emphasizes BCAAs as a key factor in performance and recovery improvement. Capsules are favored by those seeking convenience, while powders are often mixed into custom formulations for greater control. Across both forms, the majority of users report measurable benefits when BCAAs are taken consistently, especially pre- or post-exercise.

Feedback Insights

Reviewers repeatedly express surprise at the noticeable improvements BCAAs bring to their workouts, energy, and recovery. Many enter the experience skeptical, especially due to the lack of flashy marketing or the unflavored, medicinal taste of the powders, but end up converted by the actual results.

A common sentiment is feeling more "ready to go" during training sessions and recovering faster afterwards. One user shared, "I didn't feel exhausted after lifting. I even had the energy to clean my carport right after." Others describe experiencing "less soreness than expected" or being able to "push a little harder" during workouts. A long-time exerciser noted that after switching to BCAAs, they could work out more days in a row without needing rest due to soreness.

Several reviewers describe emotional and physical confidence returning: "I've never felt better," said one, while another commented, "This helps me maintain muscle and energy even with long bike commutes and demanding shifts." A vegetarian user recovering from chronic muscle weakness shared that after consistent use, they were able to reintroduce yoga and gain back strength, calling BCAAs a "life-changing" part of their routine.

Even those who disliked the bitter taste of the unflavored powders expressed strong commitment to continue using them, often citing the performance benefits as worth the effort. Phrases like "noticeable difference," "better workouts," "less fatigue," and "faster recovery" appear frequently. Some users described BCAAs as the missing link that helped them maintain progress without overreliance on stimulants or protein powders.

In summary, the emotional tone behind many reviews is one of gratitude, surprise, and renewed motivation. Users feel empowered by their ability to train harder, recover faster, and stay consistent, whether they are athletes, beginners, or simply striving to maintain strength and energy as they age.

Most Reported Benefits from Review Analysis

Branched-Chain Amino Acids (BCAAs), a combination of leucine, isoleucine, and valine, are among the most trusted supplements for those seeking support in physical performance, muscle recovery, and sustained energy. With an overall customer satisfaction rating of 4.4 out of 5 stars across thousands of reviews, users consistently describe noticeable improvements in workout endurance, faster muscle repair, and strength development.

Our analysis focused on verified positive reviews to determine which benefits are most commonly mentioned. The table below summarizes the percentage of positive reviews that cited each specific benefit. A higher percentage indicates that users frequently noticed that outcome, suggesting you may be more likely to experience similar effects if your goals align with those areas.

For example, if 40 percent of positive reviews mention improved workout performance, that means nearly half of all satisfied users reported feeling a measurable difference in their exercise capacity, stamina, or training output.

BCAA's Top Benefits Reported by Customers

BCAA's Top Benefits Reported by Customers

Benefit	%	Explanation
Workout performance	40%	Helps improve exercise output, making it easier to complete more reps, sets, or duration without hitting a wall. Often cited by users as increasing drive and sustaining intensity.
Muscle growth	22%	Supports lean muscle gain through its role in protein synthesis, particularly when used around workouts. Many users felt stronger and more toned with continued use.
Muscle recovery	19%	Aids in reducing post-workout soreness and speeds up the body's repair process, helping users bounce back faster between sessions.
Energy and endurance	16%	Helps maintain energy levels and extend physical stamina, especially during intense or long-duration training. Users often noted they could keep going when they normally would have stopped.

Benefit	%	Explanation
Fatigue reduction	3%	Minimizes feelings of exhaustion after exercise, supporting more consistent performance throughout the week. Some users described this as a "second wind" or feeling "less drained."

How to Use This Table

This table reflects what real customers most frequently noticed while using BCAAs. If your primary goal is to improve your workout performance, the data suggests you have a high likelihood of benefiting in that area, 40 percent of users who reported a positive experience mentioned this exact result. Similarly, if you're focused on building muscle or improving recovery, those benefits were also consistently reported across thousands of experiences.

Because individual results can vary based on workout intensity, diet, and overall health, these insights should be used as a guide rather than a guarantee. However, they offer a realistic and helpful snapshot of what most users experienced when incorporating BCAAs into their fitness routines.

Isoleucine

Isoleucine is one of the three branched-chain amino acids (BCAAs), alongside leucine and valine, that are essential for maintaining optimal health and enhancing physical performance. As an essential amino acid, your body cannot produce isoleucine on its own, necessitating its intake through diet or supplementation. Isoleucine plays a pivotal role in muscle metabolism, energy production, blood sugar regulation, and immune function. Whether you are an athlete striving for peak performance, someone looking to maintain lean muscle mass, or simply seeking to boost your overall vitality, isoleucine offers a range of benefits that can transform your self-care routine and elevate your quality of life.

Science-Informed Isoleucine Benefits

Isoleucine, a vital branched-chain amino acid (BCAA), plays a pivotal role in muscle health, energy regulation, and metabolic processes. Its comprehensive benefits extend to immune support and overall vitality, making it an essential supplement for those seeking enhanced physical and mental well-being.

Supports Muscle Health and Recovery

Isoleucine plays a key role in muscle protein turnover, contributing to both the repair and preservation of muscle tissue. It assists in rebuilding muscle fibers that experience stress from physical exertion and helps maintain muscle mass during periods of reduced calorie intake or intense training. This makes it a useful nutrient for those managing age-related muscle decline, recovering from physical strain, or seeking to maintain lean body composition.

Helps Regulate Energy and Endurance

Isoleucine is involved in glucose uptake within muscle cells, providing a readily available source of fuel during exercise and other forms of physical activity. By supporting efficient energy use, it may help reduce sensations of fatigue and promote longer-lasting stamina. This benefit is especially relevant for those engaged in endurance training, demanding work routines, or active lifestyles that require sustained energy throughout the day.

Contributes to Blood Sugar Stability

Some research suggests that isoleucine may influence how the body utilizes carbohydrates, contributing to more stable blood sugar levels. It may play a supportive role in glucose metabolism by enhancing the responsiveness of cells to insulin. While not a treatment for blood sugar disorders, this effect may benefit individuals who are seeking nutritional strategies to complement overall metabolic balance.

Supports Immune System Function

Isoleucine is also involved in the synthesis and repair of immune cells and tissues. It contributes to the maintenance of the body's defense systems, especially during times of stress, recovery from illness, or physical overexertion. Its presence in adequate amounts helps ensure that the body has the resources needed to mount a healthy immune response and recover efficiently from minor injuries or strain.

Encourages Healthy Skin, Hair, and Nails

As a building block of structural proteins like keratin, isoleucine supports the strength and resilience of hair and nails. It also contributes to skin health by aiding in tissue regeneration and maintaining elasticity. When nutritional intake is lacking or the body is under stress, having sufficient isoleucine may help support the repair of skin and the appearance of healthy, well-nourished hair and nails.

May Assist with Mental Focus and Mood Balance

Isoleucine is involved in the production of neurotransmitters, which influence mood, mental clarity, and concentration. While its effects are indirect, it may support brain function by contributing to a balanced neurochemical environment. This makes it a potentially helpful addition to wellness routines aimed at supporting cognitive performance and emotional resilience under stress.

Customer-Validated BCAA Benefits

L-Leucine, Isoleucine, and Valine are most commonly used together in the form of Branched-Chain Amino Acids (BCAAs), rather than as standalone supplements. While each amino acid plays a distinct role, Leucine supports muscle protein synthesis, Isoleucine helps regulate energy and blood sugar, and Valine contributes to endurance and recovery, they are typically consumed in a 2:1:1 or 3:1:1 ratio to optimize their combined effects. Because most users take BCAAs as a blend, individual reviews rarely isolate the benefits of one specific amino acid. Therefore, analyzing BCAAs collectively provides a more accurate and practical view of how users experience their real-world impact on muscle recovery, physical performance, and energy levels.

Please refer to the Customer-Reported BCAA Benefits section in the L-Leucine chapter for a comprehensive summary.

Valine

Valine is an essential amino acid and one of the three branched-chain amino acids (BCAAs), alongside leucine and isoleucine. As the body cannot synthesize valine on its own, it must be obtained through diet or supplementation. Valine plays a key role in muscle metabolism, energy regulation, immune system support, and tissue repair. Whether you are an athlete aiming to enhance performance, someone working to maintain lean muscle mass, or simply seeking to improve daily vitality, valine contributes meaningfully to both physical and mental well-being.

Science-Informed Valine Benefits

Muscle Health and Recovery

Valine supports muscle protein synthesis, which helps repair and rebuild muscle fibers after physical exertion. It also plays a protective role in preventing the breakdown of muscle tissue during periods of stress, calorie restriction, or intense training. By helping preserve lean mass and supporting muscle regeneration, valine contributes to long-term muscle function and recovery.

Valine may be supportive in cases of muscle atrophy, post-surgical rehabilitation, sarcopenia, or exercise-related muscle stress.

Energy Regulation

Valine assists in maintaining steady energy levels by promoting glucose uptake into muscle cells. This ensures the body has a readily available energy source during physical activity and can help reduce the onset of fatigue. Its role in fueling muscular endurance is especially beneficial for athletes and active individuals engaging in extended or high-intensity exercise.

Valine may be relevant for individuals facing chronic fatigue, low energy, or those seeking to improve endurance.

Cognitive Function

Valine supports the synthesis of neurotransmitters that regulate mental clarity, focus, and emotional balance. This cognitive support can enhance productivity, reduce brain fog, and improve overall concentration during mentally demanding tasks.

Valine may be beneficial for those experiencing mental fatigue, difficulty concentrating, or performance-related cognitive strain.

Immune Support

Valine contributes to immune cell production and tissue repair, helping to strengthen the body's natural defenses. It also plays a role in accelerating recovery from injuries or physical stress by supporting immune system resilience.

Valine may offer additional support for individuals prone to infections, healing slowly from injuries, or under physical or environmental stress.

Skin and Hair Health

Valine helps maintain the health of skin, hair, and nails by supporting the production of keratin, a structural protein essential for their strength and resilience. It also aids in the repair of damaged skin and promotes elasticity, contributing to a healthier and more youthful appearance.

Valine may be helpful for those experiencing brittle nails, hair thinning, or skin repair challenges.

Metabolic Regulation

Valine assists in stabilizing blood sugar levels and may help improve insulin sensitivity, supporting overall metabolic balance. Additionally, it contributes to the breakdown of fats for energy, which can assist with healthy body composition and weight management goals.

Valine may be useful for individuals addressing insulin resistance, metabolic health, or related concerns.

Customer-Reported BCAA Benefits

L-Leucine, Isoleucine, and Valine are most commonly used together as Branched-Chain Amino Acids (BCAAs) rather than taken individually. While each amino acid offers distinct benefits, leucine supports muscle protein synthesis, isoleucine contributes to energy regulation, and valine enhances physical endurance, they are typically combined in a 2:1:1 or 3:1:1 ratio for optimal synergy and effectiveness. Because most users consume BCAAs as a blend, customer reviews rarely isolate the effects of each component. As a result, evaluating real-world experiences at the combined BCAA level offers a more accurate and practical understanding of their reported benefits.

Please refer to the Leucine chapter for the Customer-Reported BCAA Benefits section.

Threonine

Threonine is an essential amino acid that plays a fundamental role in supporting overall health and maintaining the integrity of vital bodily systems. As a key building block of proteins, it contributes to the formation and function of connective tissues, muscles, and protective barriers in the body. Because the human body cannot synthesize threonine on its own, it must be obtained through dietary sources or supplementation. Its wide-ranging physiological roles include supporting immune defenses, aiding in digestive lining maintenance, and promoting the structural health of skin, hair, and nails. Whether your focus is enhancing daily wellness, optimizing recovery, or maintaining youthful vitality, threonine offers support across multiple areas of health.

Science-Informed Threonine Benefits

Muscle Health and Protein Synthesis

Threonine is critical for the formation of structural proteins such as collagen, elastin, and contractile muscle fibers. It supports muscle maintenance and repair by contributing to protein synthesis, a process essential for rebuilding tissues after physical activity. This makes threonine especially important for those recovering from exertion, managing age-related muscle loss, or seeking to preserve lean body mass during periods of caloric restriction.

Threonine may support individuals facing muscle breakdown, post-exercise fatigue, or decreased strength due to aging.

Immune System Support

Threonine contributes to a healthy immune response by supporting the synthesis of antibodies and enhancing the function of key immune cells. This amino acid plays a role in helping the body respond efficiently to everyday immune challenges and in maintaining immune vigilance under stress.

Threonine may be beneficial for those seeking to strengthen their immune resilience or who experience recurring immune strain.

Digestive Tract Integrity

As a key component in the production of mucin, threonine helps maintain the protective mucus lining that shields the gastrointestinal tract. This lining is vital for maintaining gut barrier function, optimizing nutrient absorption, and protecting against external irritants.

Threonine may support digestive comfort and overall gut health in those concerned with gut lining integrity or nutrient assimilation.

Skin, Hair, and Nail Support

Threonine contributes to the body's ability to synthesize collagen, elastin, and keratin, proteins essential for maintaining firm skin, strong hair, and resilient nails. By supporting tissue structure and elasticity, threonine plays a role in preserving a healthy, youthful appearance.

Threonine may be helpful for individuals interested in promoting radiant skin, improving hair texture, or reinforcing nail strength.

Cognitive and Emotional Balance

This amino acid is involved in neurotransmitter regulation and supports the healthy transmission of signals in the brain. Through its influence on central nervous system function, threonine contributes to emotional balance, cognitive focus, and mental clarity.

Threonine may assist individuals who are seeking to support stress resilience, emotional wellness, or sustained concentration.

Liver Function and Detoxification

Threonine helps support the liver's natural detoxification pathways by contributing to the synthesis of compounds involved in neutralizing and processing metabolic byproducts. It also plays a role in lipid metabolism, helping to maintain a balanced internal environment.

Threonine may be of interest to those focused on liver support or maintaining healthy metabolic function.

Customer-Reported Threonine Benefits

Threonine is rarely taken as a standalone supplement and is instead found in essential amino acid (EAA) blends, protein powders, and collagen-supporting formulas. As a key amino acid for protein synthesis, joint health, and skin repair, it works best alongside other amino acids like Glycine and Proline. Since consumer demand for standalone Threonine is low, there are limited user reviews to analyze. For this reason, we do not conduct a customer-validated benefits analysis and instead consider Threonine within the broader context of essential amino acid supplementation.

Histidine

Histidine is an essential amino acid that plays a fundamental role in supporting both physical health and overall vitality. As one of the key building blocks of proteins, histidine contributes to a wide range of biological functions, including the synthesis of enzymes, neurotransmitters, and cellular components that are vital for tissue maintenance and repair. Because the body cannot produce histidine on its own, it must be obtained through diet or supplementation. From supporting immune resilience to contributing to skin health and cognitive clarity, histidine offers multidimensional support for those seeking to optimize their wellness routines through targeted, science-informed nutrition.

Science-Informed Histidine Benefits

Immune System Support

Histidine contributes to the body's immune readiness by supporting the production of antibodies and helping to regulate histamine levels. Histamine plays a complex role in immune signaling, inflammation control, and allergic responses. By helping the body maintain a balanced histamine response, histidine supports both immune vigilance and inflammatory regulation.

Histidine may be beneficial for individuals seeking to support immune balance during seasonal changes, reduce environmental sensitivity, or maintain overall immune health.

Antioxidant Activity and Cellular Protection

Histidine is a biological precursor to carnosine, a dipeptide known for its antioxidant properties. Carnosine plays a role in neutralizing free radicals, protecting cells from oxidative stress, and preserving tissue integrity over time. This antioxidant capacity helps support healthy aging and cellular resilience.

Histidine may offer support to those focused on long-term cellular health and seeking to mitigate the effects of oxidative stress from environmental and lifestyle factors.

Cognitive Clarity and Neurotransmitter Support

As a precursor to histamine in the central nervous system, histidine contributes to neurotransmitter signaling involved in wakefulness, attention, appetite regulation, and emotional balance. Through its influence on brain chemistry, histidine supports mental clarity, mood stability, and cognitive performance.

Histidine may be of interest to those seeking to enhance focus, maintain mental alertness, or support emotional equilibrium during periods of high cognitive demand.

Skin, Hair, and Nail Integrity

Histidine plays a role in the synthesis of structural proteins such as collagen and keratin, which are essential for maintaining the strength and appearance of skin, hair, and nails. These proteins help retain skin elasticity, reduce signs of aging, and reinforce the resilience of hair and nails.

Histidine may be a helpful addition to the wellness routines of individuals looking to promote youthful skin, healthy hair growth, or improved nail strength.

Digestive Tract Health

This amino acid contributes to the maintenance of the mucosal lining of the gastrointestinal tract, which serves as a protective barrier for digestive tissues. By supporting gut lining integrity, histidine may assist with healthy digestion and nutrient absorption.

Histidine may be supportive for individuals seeking to promote a balanced digestive environment or address occasional digestive discomfort related to gut lining function.

Metabolic and Circulatory Function

Histidine is involved in the production of hemoglobin, the oxygen-carrying component of red blood cells. This role supports efficient oxygen transport and contributes to energy metabolism. In addition, histidine plays a role in glucose metabolism and supports metabolic balance.

Histidine may offer support to those experiencing occasional fatigue, interested in enhancing endurance, or looking to maintain healthy metabolic function.

Customer-Reported Histidine Benefits

Histidine is rarely taken as a standalone supplement and is primarily found in essential amino acid (EAA) blends or protein-rich diets. While it plays key roles in histamine production, immune function, and hemoglobin synthesis, it does not have strong consumer demand for isolated supplementation. Since standalone Histidine supplements are uncommon, there are limited user reviews to analyze. For this reason, we do not conduct a customer-validated benefits analysis or include success stories, instead considering Histidine within the broader context of essential amino acids (EAAs) and metabolic support.

EAA: Why You Need Them All Together

Essential amino acids (EAAs) are the fundamental components of proteins and play a vital role in nearly every biological function, from muscle repair and immune defense to neurotransmitter balance and skin regeneration. Although individual amino acids like lysine or tryptophan are known for their specific benefits, taking all nine essential amino acids together provides a more comprehensive and effective approach to supporting overall health and optimizing protein synthesis.

EAAs work in concert, and a deficiency in any one of them can limit the effectiveness of the others. This balance is crucial for enabling the body to repair tissue, generate energy, regulate metabolism, and support resilience under physical or emotional stress. While targeted supplementation of individual amino acids may be beneficial in specific cases, a full-spectrum EAA formula ensures the body has the complete foundation it needs for optimal daily function.

Science-Informed Essential Amino Acids Benefits

Essential amino acids include histidine, isoleucine, leucine, lysine, methionine, phenylalanine, threonine, tryptophan, and valine. Since the body cannot synthesize these amino acids on its own, they must be obtained through dietary intake or supplementation. Unlike branched-chain amino acids (BCAAs), which contain only three amino acids, EAAs provide the full range needed to support vital physiological processes across systems.

Supports Muscle Protein Synthesis and Growth

Muscle protein synthesis requires all nine essential amino acids, not just leucine or other BCAAs. Leucine initiates the mTOR pathway, which acts as the trigger for muscle building, but without the other EAAs, protein assembly cannot proceed efficiently. Supplementing with a complete EAA blend ensures that the body has all the necessary materials to support muscle repair, preserve lean body mass, and build strength. This is especially important during periods of fasting, caloric restriction, intense training, or age-related muscle loss.

Enhances Athletic Performance and Physical Recovery

During exercise, muscle fibers experience microscopic damage that must be repaired for growth and adaptation to occur. EAAs provide the raw materials needed for tissue repair, while BCAAs like isoleucine and valine offer additional fuel to delay fatigue and support endurance. Lysine and methionine play supportive roles in collagen formation and protein turnover, which are critical for restoring muscle integrity after strenuous activity. Regular supplementation with EAAs has been associated with reduced muscle soreness, faster recovery times, and improved training outcomes over time.

Supports Metabolism and Energy Production

Several EAAs contribute directly to the body's metabolic efficiency and energy balance. Threonine and methionine support the liver's ability to break down fats and process toxins, while isoleucine aids in the regulation of blood sugar and the steady release of energy. These amino acids assist in maintaining energy levels during physical exertion and reduce the risk of fatigue associated with nutrient depletion. EAAs are particularly helpful for individuals looking to optimize endurance, manage body composition, and sustain consistent energy throughout the day.

Promotes Cognitive Function and Neurotransmitter Balance

Certain essential amino acids serve as precursors to key neurotransmitters that influence mood, motivation, sleep, and mental clarity. Tryptophan supports serotonin production, which plays a central role in emotional regulation and sleep quality. Phenylalanine is used to produce dopamine and norepinephrine, two neurotransmitters that help regulate attention, focus, and alertness. Adequate intake of EAAs helps maintain cognitive balance and supports sharper thinking and more stable emotional responses during times of stress or mental fatigue.

Strengthens Immune Function and Cellular Repair

The immune system relies on essential amino acids for the production of antibodies, immune-signaling molecules, and enzymes that protect the body from illness. Histidine is particularly important for regulating immune responses and supporting red blood cell function, while lysine aids in collagen synthesis and wound healing. Together, EAAs contribute to faster recovery from infections, support tissue regeneration, and enhance the body's resilience to stressors such as illness or physical strain.

Supports Hormonal Balance and Detoxification Pathways

Essential amino acids also play a role in regulating hormones, supporting enzyme activity, and enabling detoxification processes that maintain homeostasis. Methionine is vital for liver detoxification and for the production of glutathione, a powerful antioxidant that protects cells from oxidative stress. Phenylalanine and lysine contribute to the synthesis of hormones that regulate the thyroid, adrenal function, and neurological signaling. By supporting hormonal regulation and metabolic detoxification, EAAs contribute to a more stable and balanced internal environment.

Why Supplementing with EAAs Can Be Essential

Because the body cannot make essential amino acids on its own, a consistent and adequate dietary supply is necessary to maintain muscle health, brain function, immune resilience, and overall well-being. Unfortunately, many modern diets lack sufficient EAAs due to low protein quality or restricted intake. Supplementation can help fill these gaps and provide the body with the full complement of amino acids it needs to function efficiently.

Unlike single amino acid products, which only target specific needs, full-spectrum EAA formulas offer a comprehensive solution that supports multiple body systems. Whether your goal is to improve recovery, maintain strength, support mental clarity, or enhance daily energy levels, supplementing with all nine essential amino acids ensures that your body receives the foundational support it needs to thrive.

Customer-Reported Essential Amino Acid Benefits

Essential Amino Acids (EAAs) are highly valued by users for their ability to support recovery, energy, and physical performance, especially when dietary protein intake is limited or inconsistent. With a strong customer rating of 4.5 out of 5 stars across thousands of reviews, these supplements have become a cornerstone in many people's self-care routines. Users consistently report improved muscle recovery, increased energy, enhanced stamina, and noticeable differences in hair, skin, and mood. Whether taken to support athletic goals, manage age-related muscle concerns, or complement a low-protein diet, EAAs appear to deliver meaningful results for a wide range of individuals.

Use Case Patterns Observed

Many people use EAAs as part of a fitness or recovery routine, especially those who engage in regular strength training, cardio, or endurance sports. Users often take them before or after workouts to speed up muscle repair, reduce soreness, and maintain lean body mass. They are also frequently used by individuals over the age of 40 who want to preserve muscle, boost energy, or support graceful aging.

Some reviewers with limited protein intake, due to vegetarian or low-calorie diets, use EAAs to fill nutritional gaps without relying on large amounts of food or protein shakes. Others turn to EAAs for recovery support following surgery, illness, or fatigue, often alongside other supplements like collagen, glutamine, or hyaluronic acid. A number of users take EAAs in the morning on an empty stomach or in split doses throughout the day to maintain energy and mental clarity.

Feedback Insights

Customers often express genuine surprise and enthusiasm about the benefits they experience from taking EAAs. Many describe a noticeable reduction in muscle soreness, with several stating they "recovered faster" or "felt less drained" after workouts. Some who were previously dealing with chronic fatigue or post-exercise crashes shared that EAAs gave them a renewed sense of stamina, using words like "energized," "stronger," and "motivated." A number of users over the age of 50 noted that the supplements helped them stay consistent with their exercise routines, even after decades of training.

Physical transformation is a recurring theme. People describe feeling stronger, seeing visible muscle definition, and even losing stubborn weight. One reviewer shared that they felt "less hungry and more active," while others mentioned an improved sense of well-being, both mentally and physically. Those recovering from surgery or injury found that EAAs helped support their healing and strength-building efforts during the recovery process. Several noted improvements in hair thickness, nail strength, and skin health, describing these changes as unexpected but welcome benefits.

One reviewer summed it up simply: "This product changed my life. I feel better, stronger, and finally able to stay active again."

Most Reported Benefits from Review Analysis

To better understand how people experience Essential Amino Acids (EAAs) in real life, we conducted an in-depth analysis of verified customer reviews, focusing on the benefits most frequently mentioned by satisfied users. The table below reflects the distribution of reported effects across thousands of positive reviews. While individual responses can vary, a higher percentage suggests a more consistent trend among users.

For example, 36% of reviewers specifically highlighted improvements in workout performance, indicating that if you're seeking better exercise output or physical endurance, EAAs may be a valuable option to consider. Energy enhancement and muscle recovery were also frequently mentioned, suggesting that these amino acids support both immediate performance and longer-term progress.

Below is a summary table of EAAs' top benefits as reported by customers:

Benefit	%	Explanation
Workout Performance	36%	Users commonly report improved strength, stamina, and workout intensity, often describing smoother training sessions and better physical output.
Energy and Endurance	35%	Many feel a sustained boost in daily energy, with less fatigue during physical or mental activity. This benefit is often mentioned by those with demanding routines.
Muscle Recovery	20%	A large portion of reviewers note faster recovery after workouts, with less soreness and quicker return to normal activity.
Muscle Growth	6%	Some users mention improved muscle tone and lean mass, especially when paired with consistent exercise and protein intake.
Cognitive Function	3%	A smaller group reports increased mental clarity, focus, and motivation, particularly when EAAs are used regularly in the morning or before workouts.

How to Use This Guide

If you're considering EAAs to support your physical performance, boost energy, or recover more efficiently, this guide provides a practical view into what other users are experiencing most often. These percentages do not guarantee specific outcomes, but they highlight the patterns that show up consistently across real-world feedback.

It's worth noting that many people report experiencing more than one benefit at the same time, and the most noticeable improvements often emerge after several weeks of steady use. Whether your goals include fitness, vitality, or everyday stamina, EAAs are praised for delivering reliable support without unnecessary additives or complications.

With a high average satisfaction rating and a wide range of reported benefits, EAAs continue to earn their place as a trusted daily supplement for individuals looking to stay strong, energized, and resilient.

Using Essential Amino Acids

Convenient Capsule or Powder Use

Essential amino acids (EAAs) are available in both capsule and powder form, making it easy to fit into different lifestyles and routines. Capsules offer a convenient, pre-measured solution for those who need a quick, no-fuss option, especially useful for busy schedules or travel. Powdered EAAs, in contrast, allow for flexible dosing and can be easily mixed with water, smoothies, or post-exercise shakes, providing rapid absorption and personalized control over intake.

No matter which form you choose, supplementing EAAs helps ensure your body receives a full complement of essential nutrients that may not always be present in ideal amounts through diet alone. While capsules are ideal for consistent daily use, powders may be preferred by individuals seeking higher doses or a more tailored approach.

Dosage and Timing Recommendations

Essential amino acids (EAAs) can be used to support a variety of health goals, including daily wellness, physical performance, and recovery. The appropriate amount may vary depending on individual needs, lifestyle, and health status.

For general wellness, many people choose to take EAAs regularly to help maintain nutrient balance and support metabolic function. Those with more intensive needs—such as athletes, or individuals recovering from physical stress, illness, or surgery—may find that a more targeted or consistent approach works best.

Always refer to the serving guidelines provided on your product's label. If you have specific health concerns or are considering EAAs for therapeutic purposes, consulting a qualified healthcare provider is the best way to determine the right strategy for your needs.

Timing Tips

Post-exercise: Consuming EAAs immediately after a workout may help promote muscle repair, reduce soreness, and support recovery.

Morning or pre-workout: Taking EAAs before the start of your day or physical activity may help improve energy, stamina, and mental clarity.

During fasting: EAAs can be used during fasting periods to help preserve lean muscle and support energy without breaking the fast.

If you are using an individual amino acid for a specific need, follow the product's instructions or seek advice from a healthcare practitioner for optimal results and safety.

Safety and Precautions

EAAs are generally considered safe when used as directed. However, because amino acids are processed through the liver and kidneys, individuals with known liver or kidney conditions should consult their healthcare provider before starting supplementation.

To ensure the best results, choose high-quality products from trusted manufacturers that use third-party testing to verify purity and potency. Taking the time to select the right supplement can help you experience the full benefits that EAAs have to offer, naturally and effectively.

N-Acetyl Cysteine (NAC)

N-Acetyl Cysteine, often abbreviated as NAC, is a stable, supplement form of the amino acid cysteine. It is best known for its role in supporting antioxidant defenses, promoting detoxification, and maintaining respiratory and neurological health. NAC is particularly valued for its ability to help replenish glutathione, the body's most powerful antioxidant, which plays a central role in cellular protection, repair, and immune balance.

As a versatile compound, NAC is used by a wide range of individuals seeking support for vitality, mental focus, lung function, reproductive wellness, and detox pathways. Since the body cannot produce NAC on its own, it must be obtained through supplementation. When used appropriately, it may offer broad support for health maintenance, especially under modern-day stressors and environmental exposures.

Science-Informed NAC Benefits

Antioxidant Defense and Cellular Protection

NAC is best known for its ability to promote the synthesis of glutathione, a compound that defends cells against oxidative stress and supports cellular repair. Glutathione is involved in hundreds of enzymatic processes in the body and is considered one of the most critical molecules for maintaining long-term health. By supporting glutathione production, NAC may help protect tissues from oxidative damage and assist in healthy aging and recovery. This function has made NAC a popular choice among those concerned with fatigue, brain fog, and maintaining cognitive and cardiovascular health over time.

Detoxification and Liver Support

NAC contributes to healthy detoxification by supporting the liver's natural processes for neutralizing and eliminating toxins. It plays a particularly important role in helping the body manage exposure to environmental pollutants, medications, and metabolic byproducts. In clinical settings, NAC is used to support the liver during toxic overload, and in everyday use, it is commonly chosen by individuals seeking to maintain long-term liver wellness or promote efficient metabolism.

Respiratory Health and Airway Comfort

One of NAC's distinguishing features is its mucolytic effect, the ability to help break down and thin mucus. This supports easier breathing and helps clear the airways, especially in conditions associated with congestion or inflammation. NAC also has antioxidant properties that benefit lung tissues, making it a well-regarded option for those who want to support seasonal respiratory resilience or maintain healthy breathing function year-round.

Cognitive Function and Emotional Balance

NAC may also play a role in supporting brain health. It influences levels of glutamate, a neurotransmitter involved in learning, memory, and mood regulation. In this way, NAC contributes to emotional balance and mental clarity. It is often chosen by individuals looking for support with focus, mood steadiness, or occasional mental fatigue. Its antioxidant action also helps protect brain cells from the effects of oxidative stress, which can impact long-term cognitive wellness.

Immune System Support

Through its antioxidant and anti-inflammatory mechanisms, NAC plays a supporting role in immune resilience. By promoting glutathione production and reducing cellular stress, it helps maintain a balanced immune response. Many individuals take NAC during times of immune vulnerability or seasonal transitions to reinforce their body's natural defenses.

Reproductive and Fertility Support

NAC is increasingly studied for its role in supporting reproductive wellness. Its antioxidant properties may help protect reproductive tissues from oxidative damage, and it has been used to support healthy ovarian and sperm function. While individual results vary, NAC is commonly included in protocols aimed at maintaining reproductive health in both men and women.

Digestive and Gut Integrity

The gastrointestinal tract relies on a healthy mucosal lining to absorb nutrients and protect against irritants. NAC has been shown to support this protective barrier by promoting mucosal balance and managing oxidative stress in the gut. Some individuals report improved digestive comfort and regularity when using NAC as part of a broader approach to gut wellness.

Thyroid Health and Metabolic Support

Oxidative stress is thought to play a role in many thyroid-related concerns. NAC's ability to reduce this stress and support the body's detoxification pathways makes it a promising tool for maintaining thyroid balance. While not a replacement for thyroid medication,

NAC is sometimes used alongside a wellness plan aimed at supporting energy, metabolism, and hormonal regulation.

Customer-Reported NAC Benefits

With a remarkable 4.6 out of 5 average rating and thousands of detailed reviews, N-Acetyl Cysteine (NAC) has become a trusted and widely used supplement for those seeking support in energy, mental clarity, mood balance, respiratory health, and immune resilience. Our analysis of verified customer experiences reveals not just the breadth of NAC's impact, but also the emotional weight behind those transformations. From individuals navigating intense life stress or chronic health struggles to those simply looking to feel better and stay well, NAC has left a lasting impression on diverse users.

Use Case Patterns Observed

Many people turn to NAC after struggling with ongoing fatigue, mental fog, chronic inflammation, or recurring respiratory issues. A significant number mention discovering NAC as part of a deeper search for natural wellness solutions when conventional treatments fell short or introduced unwanted side effects. Others adopt NAC as part of a broader detox or longevity strategy, especially after learning about its relationship to glutathione production, the body's most important antioxidant. Several reviewers specifically mention using NAC in combination with glycine or magnesium to enhance its effects, particularly for mental clarity, mood regulation, or metabolic recovery. NAC is also widely adopted by individuals managing symptoms associated with obsessive-compulsive tendencies, anxiety, emotional dysregulation, and addiction recovery. Parents seeking alternative approaches to support children with behavioral or mood-related concerns also report turning to NAC with cautious optimism, and in many cases, profound relief. In addition, those recovering from long-haul fatigue, immune suppression, or persistent congestion often report discovering NAC during a period of intense health reevaluation.

Feedback Insights

The emotional tone of NAC reviews is striking. Many users describe a sense of gratitude and even disbelief at the positive changes they observe, often after years of frustration with conventional approaches. One user called NAC a "lifesaver" after seeing noticeable relief from overwhelming compulsions and racing thoughts, describing how they were "left with the odd sensation of nothing that needed doing." Others echoed this shift in mental state, noting a remarkable reduction in obsessive behaviors, skin picking, or anxiety-driven habits. Reviewers often emphasize how surprised they were by the speed and depth of improvement. Phrases like "I could breathe again," "my energy came back," "my mood lifted," and "it changed my life" appear again and again, reflecting the degree of personal impact.

Several parents shared stories of children experiencing sudden breakthroughs in reading comprehension, mood, or focus within days of starting NAC, outcomes they previously thought impossible. For others, the benefit was more physical: easing of persistent coughing, less mucus production, or newfound stamina after years of respiratory discomfort. Some mentioned bouncing back from post-viral fatigue or chronic immune suppression. The recovery experiences are often described with a sense of awe and emotional relief. One user wrote about how they were able to return to running and cycling again, with joint pain and inflammation finally under control. Others remarked that NAC helped them overcome long-term hair loss, stubborn fat retention related to stress, or deeply rooted fatigue that resisted other interventions.

Even users who started NAC without clear expectations often described feeling more balanced and energized within a few weeks. A common sentiment is that NAC helped bring their body "back into alignment," and that they could finally see themselves making progress with health goals that had previously seemed unattainable. While results varied, the unifying thread across thousands of testimonials was a deep appreciation for NAC's ability to support resilience in the face of persistent health challenges, especially when other tools had fallen short.

Most Reported Benefits from Review Analysis

To understand how NAC is helping people in real-world settings, we conducted a detailed analysis of verified customer reviews, focusing on the most commonly reported benefits among satisfied users. The table below reflects the percentage of reviewers who specifically mentioned each type of improvement. While individual experiences will always vary, higher percentages indicate clear trends in how NAC is most often perceived and used.

For instance, 30% of reviewers described noticeable improvements in liver health and detoxification, suggesting that if detox support is your goal, NAC may offer especially consistent benefits. Lung and respiratory improvements were also commonly mentioned, followed closely by enhanced emotional balance, immune resilience, and clearer mental functioning. Together, these data points reveal a supplement praised not just for one single purpose, but for its broad support of whole-body well-being.

Below is a summary table of NAC's top benefits as reported by customers:

Benefit	%	Explanation
Liver Detoxification	30%	Enhances liver health by promoting glutathione production, a powerful antioxidant and detoxifier.
Lung & Respiratory Health	21%	Supports clearer breathing by thinning mucus and easing respiratory discomfort.
Mood & Stress Relief	20%	Helps regulate neurotransmitters, often described as calming mental noise and lifting mood.
Immune Support	17%	Strengthens immune defenses by reducing oxidative stress and supporting overall cellular health.
Brain & Mental Clarity	12%	Promotes focus and mental sharpness, reducing fog and improving clarity.

How to Use This Guide

If you are considering NAC to support liver detoxification, enhance your breathing, or improve emotional and cognitive well-being, these findings offer a practical reference point. The percentages shown reflect how often users voluntarily shared each benefit in their reviews, not guaranteed outcomes, but common experiences that highlight where NAC appears to be most helpful in real-world use.

Many individuals report experiencing more than one benefit at a time, especially when taking NAC consistently over several weeks or months. Whether your goal is to feel clearer, breathe easier, or regain a sense of calm and energy, these patterns can help you decide whether NAC is the right addition to your self-care strategy. Its consistently high satisfaction ratings, combined with the breadth of reported benefits, make NAC one of the most trusted and versatile amino acid-based supplements in use today.

Glutathione

Glutathione is often described as the body's "master antioxidant," a title it earns through its unique ability to defend cells from oxidative stress at the deepest levels. Composed of three amino acids, glutamine, cysteine, and glycine, glutathione is synthesized naturally in the liver and plays a pivotal role in numerous critical biological processes. Unlike many other antioxidants that operate primarily outside of cells, glutathione works from within, protecting against free radical damage, aiding in detoxification, supporting the immune system, and preserving the integrity of cellular function. Whether your focus is on maintaining vibrant health, detoxifying environmental and metabolic waste, or enhancing skin clarity and cognitive sharpness, glutathione offers a broad spectrum of support that aligns with many modern wellness goals.

Science-Informed Glutathione Benefits

Antioxidant Defense

Glutathione plays a central role in neutralizing free radicals and maintaining the body's oxidative balance. This activity protects cells from damage that accumulates through daily exposure to stress, pollution, poor diet, and aging. Glutathione's antioxidant power is particularly important for people who experience high levels of oxidative stress, whether due to environmental factors or internal imbalances. By reducing oxidative load, glutathione supports long-term health and may help mitigate risks associated with cardiovascular conditions, metabolic disorders such as diabetes, and chronic fatigue. Its presence also helps regenerate other antioxidants like vitamin C and vitamin E, making it an integral part of the body's defense network.

Detoxification Support

One of glutathione's most essential roles is in the detoxification process, particularly within the liver. It binds with heavy metals, pharmaceutical residues, and environmental pollutants, transforming them into water-soluble forms that the body can safely excrete. This process reduces toxic burden and helps the liver maintain optimal function. Individuals who are regularly exposed to chemical irritants, medications, alcohol, or industrial pollutants may find particular value in supporting their detox pathways through glutathione. Additionally, glutathione contributes to the safe breakdown and removal of metabolic waste products that, if accumulated, can contribute to fatigue and systemic inflammation.

Immune Function Regulation

Glutathione supports the immune system by enhancing the function of immune cells, including lymphocytes and natural killer cells. It plays a regulatory role in the body's inflammatory response, helping to keep inflammation in check while ensuring that defenses remain active and responsive. In conditions where immune activity is suppressed or chronically overstimulated, glutathione may help restore a more balanced response. It has been studied for its ability to support immune resilience, especially in individuals prone to frequent colds, seasonal illnesses, or low immune reactivity. Its presence may also aid in modulating autoimmune activity when immune signals become dysregulated.

Cellular Energy and Repair

At the cellular level, glutathione supports critical functions such as mitochondrial protection, DNA repair, and protein synthesis. These processes are fundamental to sustaining cellular energy and preventing long-term damage. When glutathione levels are adequate, cells are better equipped to handle daily stressors and recover from injury or fatigue. This can result in improved physical stamina, sharper mental energy, and better recovery from exertion or illness. People experiencing chronic fatigue or mitochondrial dysfunction may particularly benefit from supporting their glutathione levels to optimize energy metabolism and promote overall vitality.

Skin Radiance and Complexion

In the realm of skin health, glutathione has gained attention for its role in promoting a brighter and more even skin tone. It is known to influence melanin production, which can lead to reduced appearance of hyperpigmentation, age spots, and discoloration. As an antioxidant, it also protects skin cells from UV-related oxidative damage and environmental aging. Individuals who incorporate glutathione into their routines often report improvements in skin clarity, smoothness, and elasticity over time. Its internal support for skin renewal, combined with detoxification and inflammation reduction, offers a holistic pathway to clearer, more radiant skin.

Cognitive Support and Mental Clarity

In the brain, glutathione is essential for protecting neurons from oxidative stress and maintaining healthy neurotransmitter activity. This is especially important in aging populations or those at risk of cognitive decline. Research has explored its role in supporting brain health and slowing the progression of neurodegenerative conditions by stabilizing the cellular environment within the central nervous system. Individuals experiencing brain fog, poor concentration, or memory issues may benefit from increased glutathione availability, as it helps preserve cognitive function and sharpness. By reducing inflammation and oxidative burden in the brain, it creates a clearer and more stable mental environment.

Customer-Reported Glutathione Benefits

With an impressive average rating of 4.5 out of 5 from thousands of verified users, glutathione is celebrated for its diverse benefits, ranging from skin clarity and energy support to detoxification, cognitive well-being, and immune resilience. This powerful antioxidant is frequently praised for its noticeable effects, even among users who had previously tried multiple other supplements without success. While individual responses vary, many users consistently report improved skin appearance, brighter complexions, greater energy, emotional balance, and better overall health after regular use.

The following insights are drawn from a large body of real-world reviews, helping illustrate how people actually use glutathione and what types of experiences they most often share. These patterns do not represent guaranteed outcomes but can provide a helpful perspective if you are considering glutathione as part of your wellness plan.

Use Case Patterns Observed

People turn to glutathione for a wide range of personal health goals. One of the most prominent uses is for skin-related concerns, including dull complexion, hyperpigmentation, melasma, and acne scarring. Many users describe incorporating glutathione alongside vitamin C, exfoliants, and sun protection to support brighter, more even-toned skin. Some use it specifically to help fade dark spots or address uneven areas, while others report enhanced skin radiance even without expecting it.

Another large group takes glutathione to support detoxification and liver health, especially after prolonged stress, medication use, or alcohol exposure. Several reviewers mention long-standing liver enzyme issues or sluggishness improving over time. It is also commonly used as a complementary aid during recovery from illness or after surgery, often to help replenish antioxidant levels and support cellular resilience.

A number of users take glutathione for energy, mood, or cognitive support, especially those recovering from burnout or chronic stress. Others explore it as a tool to support immune function or promote graceful aging. Some parents use it for older family members with tremors or balance issues potentially linked to antioxidant depletion, and younger users describe a general desire to maintain vibrant health and glowing skin.

Feedback Insights

The emotional tone in glutathione reviews often shifts from cautious optimism to surprise and genuine enthusiasm. Some users admit they were skeptical at first, expecting little more than a minor supplement boost, only to be taken aback by the noticeable changes they experienced. One reviewer wrote that after just a few days, they "looked in the mirror and couldn't believe the glow," describing their complexion as refreshed and even radiant. Others reported compliments from friends or coworkers who noticed their skin becoming smoother, more even, or visibly brighter, even when the user hadn't made any other changes.

For those using glutathione for skin support, many describe a journey of experimentation, often tracking subtle improvements over weeks or months. While some users hoped for dramatic skin lightening and instead observed only gradual brightening or enhanced hydration, others were thrilled with results like fading dark elbows, reduced hyperpigmentation, or smoother texture. Even users with long-standing concerns such as melasma or post-inflammatory spots found unexpected improvements, often noting that glutathione helped where other treatments had failed.

Energy-related feedback also shows up repeatedly, with some saying they felt more motivated or alert within days of starting supplementation. One woman recovering from a difficult life chapter shared that glutathione brought her "residual energy back" and inspired her to move again, even completing workouts she had put off for months. Others described feeling more emotionally balanced, with one person noting they experienced a "subtle euphoria" that helped lift their mood and stamina.

In reviews focused on detoxification, many users report feeling "cleaner" or less weighed down, often noting better digestion, improved skin, or fewer post-alcohol symptoms. Some even found relief from long-standing aches or inflammation they hadn't connected to oxidative stress until they started supplementing. A user managing liver health explained that their bloodwork normalized after consistent glutathione use, while another shared that their hangovers all but disappeared.

For those using glutathione to support loved ones, such as elderly parents dealing with tremors or unsteadiness, the feedback is deeply personal. One reviewer said their grandmother's shaking improved within two days, something they hadn't seen with any other intervention. Moments like these reflect not just physical improvements, but also the emotional relief of watching someone regain confidence and comfort.

Across many of these reviews, people often describe glutathione as a supplement they plan to keep taking for the long haul. Whether it's clearer skin, steadier mood, or better recovery from stress, the benefits, however varied, seem to leave a lasting impression on those who experience them.

Most Reported Benefits from Review Analysis

To better understand how people are actually experiencing glutathione, we conducted a detailed analysis of verified customer reviews. This section focuses specifically on the benefits most frequently mentioned by satisfied users. The table below reflects the distribution of reported benefits across thousands of positive experiences. While individual results always vary, a higher percentage suggests a more consistent pattern of improvement observed by other users.

For example, if 40 percent of reviewers mentioned skin brightening and complexion enhancement, it suggests that individuals with similar skin-related goals may be more likely to notice visible changes over time. In the same way, reports of improved energy, detoxification, or immune support help illustrate which wellness areas glutathione may support most consistently, based on real-world use.

Glutathione's Top Benefits Reported by Customers

Benefit	%	Explanation
Skin Health & Brightening	40%	Promotes a radiant complexion, reduces dark spots, and enhances skin clarity.
Energy & Fatigue Reduction	22%	Enhances energy levels by reducing oxidative stress and improving mitochondrial function.

Benefit	%	Explanation
Liver Detoxification	17%	Supports liver function by aiding in the removal of toxins and oxidative stress.
Anti-Aging & Cellular Health	11%	Supports cellular repair, reduces oxidative damage, and promotes youthful vitality.
Immune Support	10%	Boosts the immune system by reducing inflammation and strengthening the body's defenses.

How to Use This Guide

If you are considering glutathione for a specific purpose, such as enhancing skin tone, improving energy, or supporting liver detoxification, this data provides a helpful starting point. The percentages above reflect how often users mention each benefit in their positive reviews. While they do not guarantee individual results, they offer valuable insight into the areas where users most frequently report positive outcomes.

Many individuals report experiencing multiple benefits at once, with skin clarity, fatigue reduction, and immune resilience often improving in parallel. In some cases, visible results were noted within weeks, while others saw continued improvements over several months of consistent use. As with any supplement, responses vary based on a range of personal factors including baseline health, dosage, absorption, and supporting lifestyle habits.

Whether your focus is skin renewal, deeper detoxification, or long-term wellness, glutathione continues to earn its reputation as a foundational antioxidant that supports health from the inside out.

Glycine

Glycine is the simplest amino acid in structure, but its functions within the human body are anything but simple. As a non-essential amino acid, it is naturally produced by the body, yet supplemental glycine can significantly enhance several key aspects of health and wellness. Glycine serves as a critical building block for proteins and plays essential roles in neurotransmission, detoxification, collagen formation, and cellular repair. It also supports the synthesis of other important compounds, including glutathione, creatine, and heme, making it foundational to many biological processes.

Whether your focus is on improving sleep, strengthening bones and joints, supporting brain health, or nourishing the skin from within, glycine offers a wide array of supportive benefits. Scientific studies continue to explore and confirm the vital contributions of glycine to both everyday wellness and long-term health.

Science-Informed Glycine Benefits

Supports Restful Sleep

Glycine has been shown to help promote deeper, more restorative sleep. It works by helping to lower core body temperature in the evening, a signal that helps the body transition into sleep mode. Clinical studies have demonstrated that glycine supplementation before bedtime can reduce the time it takes to fall asleep, improve sleep continuity, and enhance overall sleep satisfaction. Its calming effects on the central nervous system also make it a useful support for individuals dealing with occasional stress-related sleep disturbances or irregular sleep patterns.

Enhances Cognitive Function and Focus

In the brain, glycine functions as an inhibitory neurotransmitter, helping to modulate the excitability of nerve signals and promote a sense of calm and clarity. It supports mental performance by helping reduce overstimulation and balancing other neurotransmitters such as glutamate. Research indicates that glycine may help improve memory retention, attention, and cognitive resilience, particularly in older adults or those experiencing cognitive strain. It is being explored for its potential neuroprotective properties in age-related cognitive decline and other neurological concerns.

Promotes Joint and Bone Health

As a fundamental component of collagen, glycine plays a direct role in maintaining the strength and elasticity of connective tissues. It is involved in the structural integrity of cartilage, tendons, ligaments, and bones, all of which rely on collagen to remain strong and functional. Adequate glycine intake supports bone density and may help protect against age-related bone and joint degradation. For individuals engaged in physical activity or recovering from injury, glycine contributes to tissue repair and structural resilience.

Supports Metabolic and Muscle Health

Glycine plays an important role in metabolic regulation. It assists in the management of blood sugar levels by improving insulin sensitivity and supporting glucose metabolism. Through its role in protein synthesis, glycine also helps maintain muscle mass, especially in older adults or those with reduced physical activity. It has been studied for its potential to support healthy body composition and energy balance, particularly in the context of aging and metabolic challenges.

Contributes to Digestive Wellness

In the digestive system, glycine helps maintain the health of the gastrointestinal lining. It supports the production of protective mucus, which helps shield the stomach and intestines from irritation and inflammation. Its calming effects on the gut can contribute to improved digestion and nutrient absorption. Glycine has been studied in connection with maintaining intestinal integrity, especially in individuals with conditions affecting the gut barrier or inflammatory balance.

Nourishes Skin from Within

Glycine is one of the most abundant amino acids in the body's collagen, making it essential for skin elasticity, hydration, and regeneration. Regular intake of glycine may support smoother, firmer skin by enhancing the body's ability to repair tissues and build healthy collagen networks. It has been studied for its role in wound healing and skin renewal, and may contribute to a more even skin tone and reduced visibility of scars or blemishes. As part of a comprehensive wellness routine, glycine supports a more vibrant, youthful appearance over time.

Customer-Reported Glycine Benefits

Glycine is widely appreciated by users for its ability to support deeper sleep, calm the nervous system, and improve mood and cognitive clarity. With a strong average rating of 4.5 out of 5 stars across thousands of reviews, glycine has earned the trust of those seeking a safe, non-habit-forming way to feel more rested, relaxed, and resilient. While glycine is a naturally occurring amino acid produced by the body, many reviewers report that supplementation has made a noticeable difference in their day-to-day quality of life. For many users, this simple supplement has become an essential part of their nighttime routine and emotional wellness toolkit.

Use Case Patterns Observed

The majority of reviewers report taking glycine to improve sleep, especially when dealing with trouble falling asleep, waking up too early, or getting insufficient deep rest. Some users began with glycine after trying multiple other supplements or medications with limited success, while others added it to their nighttime routine based on research, podcast recommendations, or healthcare provider advice. Many people paired glycine with other calming nutrients like magnesium, GABA, or melatonin, though a significant number mentioned that glycine alone made a meaningful difference. A smaller but notable group used glycine for anxiety, stress, or nervous system support during the day, while a few reported broader wellness benefits such as better focus, reduced fatigue, and overall cognitive clarity. A handful of users also shared experiences related to hormonal changes, hot flashes, or detoxification support.

Feedback Insights

Reviewers often describe glycine as a surprising discovery, calling it "life-changing," "a game-changer," and "the best sleep support I've ever tried." Many express a deep sense of gratitude and relief, especially those who had struggled with poor sleep for years. One user shared that after decades of insomnia, glycine finally helped them sleep through the night without feeling groggy in the morning. Another described the emotional impact of waking up well-rested, saying it improved their productivity, mood, and general outlook on life. Several users tracked their sleep data using wearable devices and noticed measurable increases in deep sleep. Others mentioned how glycine helped them wake up less often, fall back asleep more easily, and feel more refreshed the next day.

The emotional tone across reviews is often one of hope, surprise, and empowerment. People speak of glycine as gentle yet effective, with comments like "I sleep like a baby," "I feel calmer and clearer," and "finally something that actually works." Some even shared that glycine helped their spouse, teenager, or pet find better rest and balance. For those who had tried numerous approaches without lasting success, glycine offered a simple, affordable solution that felt both safe and impactful. While not every user experienced dramatic results, the overall sentiment was overwhelmingly positive, with many noting that glycine is now a permanent part of their daily routine.

Most Reported Benefits from Review Analysis

Glycine is a foundational amino acid that supports sleep, cognitive health, and overall physical recovery. Based on thousands of user reviews and an impressive average rating of 4.5 out of 5 stars, glycine is consistently praised for helping people feel calmer, sleep more deeply, and function more clearly during the day. While it naturally occurs in the body, many users turn to supplementation for additional support, especially when daily stress, poor sleep, or age-related changes start to interfere with rest and vitality.

Our analysis of positive customer feedback reveals the most commonly reported benefits of glycine. These percentages reflect how often each outcome was mentioned among reviewers who experienced noticeable improvements. The higher the percentage, the more frequently that benefit was cited by satisfied users. This data can help guide your expectations and highlight the types of benefits glycine may support based on real-world experiences.

Glycine's Top Benefits Reported by Customers

Benefit	%	Explanation
Sleep Quality & Relaxation	85%	Supports deep, uninterrupted sleep and promotes relaxation by calming the nervous system.
Cognitive Function & Memory	7%	Enhances focus, supports mental clarity, and improves memory retention.
Muscle Growth & Recovery	4%	Aids in muscle repair, reduces soreness, and supports post-exercise recovery.
Skin & Anti-Aging Benefits	2%	Promotes skin elasticity, supports collagen production, and encourages youthful appearance.
Joint & Connective Tissue Health	1%	Supports joint comfort and helps maintain the structure of connective tissues.

How to Use This Table

This table summarizes how real users describe their experiences with glycine, highlighting the areas where it is most often reported to help. While everyone's body responds differently, these trends can give you a sense of what others have found most noticeable and impactful. If your primary goal is to sleep better, for example, glycine may be especially promising given the overwhelming number of reviewers who report improvements in sleep quality and relaxation. Benefits in areas like cognitive support, skin health, and recovery may be more subtle or take longer to observe, but many users still find them meaningful over time.

These insights are based on personal experiences shared in public reviews and should not be interpreted as medical advice or guarantees of effect. As always, consider consulting a healthcare professional to determine whether glycine is appropriate for your specific needs and health goals.

Tyrosine

Tyrosine is a non-essential amino acid that plays an essential role in maintaining physical and mental balance, especially during times of increased demand. While the body can produce tyrosine from phenylalanine, a variety of stressors, whether physical, emotional, or environmental, can elevate the body's need for this important nutrient. Tyrosine acts as a biochemical building block, supporting the synthesis of neurotransmitters, thyroid hormones, and structural proteins that keep key systems in the body functioning smoothly.

Individuals often turn to tyrosine to support mental performance, stress management, energy levels, and metabolic stability. It is commonly used by students, professionals, athletes, and those navigating demanding schedules or emotionally taxing periods. From enhancing focus under pressure to promoting a sense of balance during fatigue, tyrosine offers broad support for those seeking to maintain clarity, resilience, and physical vitality as part of a proactive wellness routine.

Science-Informed Tyrosine Benefits

Cognitive Performance

Tyrosine contributes to the synthesis of neurotransmitters such as dopamine, norepinephrine, and epinephrine, which regulate alertness, concentration, and mental stamina. Under stressful or cognitively demanding conditions, these neurotransmitters can become depleted, leading to feelings of mental fog or fatigue. Tyrosine helps support the brain's ability to maintain focus and clarity, particularly in situations involving sleep deprivation, multitasking, or emotional stress. Many people find that supplementation helps them stay mentally sharp and productive during intense periods of work or study.

Stress Support

One of tyrosine's most notable roles is in supporting the body's stress response. By helping maintain neurotransmitter balance, tyrosine can assist the nervous system in adapting to both acute and chronic stress. When the brain is under pressure, the need for dopamine and norepinephrine rises. Tyrosine helps the body keep up with this increased demand, promoting greater emotional steadiness and a more balanced response to daily challenges.

Thyroid Hormone Production

Tyrosine serves as a precursor to the thyroid hormones T3 and T4, which are essential regulators of metabolism, body temperature, and energy output. Along with iodine, tyrosine is needed to produce these hormones efficiently. Supplementing with tyrosine may offer support for individuals who are seeking to maintain healthy thyroid function, especially when energy levels or metabolic balance feel off despite good lifestyle habits.

Metabolic and Physical Endurance

Because it contributes to both neurotransmitter and hormone synthesis, tyrosine also plays a role in energy balance and physical performance. It is sometimes used as part of fitness or recovery routines to help reduce fatigue and maintain stamina during exercise or physically demanding tasks. Those with active lifestyles may benefit from its support in sustaining consistent energy output and post-exertion recovery.

Skin and Hair Vitality

Tyrosine supports melanin production, which contributes to hair and skin pigmentation. It also aids in the synthesis of collagen and other structural proteins that promote skin elasticity and hair strength. While tyrosine is not used as a cosmetic, its internal support for skin and hair structure makes it a valuable addition for individuals focused on long-term vitality and visible health.

Cardiovascular Function

The catecholamines synthesized from tyrosine influence heart rate, blood vessel tone, and the body's adaptive response to stress. Tyrosine's support of these pathways may contribute to better cardiovascular efficiency during physical activity or mental exertion. Individuals aiming to support heart health as part of a larger wellness routine may find tyrosine a useful nutritional ally.

Motor Coordination and Neuromuscular Support

Tyrosine's influence on dopamine also has implications for neuromuscular signaling and coordination. Adequate dopamine levels are essential for smooth, purposeful movement and physical control. Tyrosine is sometimes used by individuals who want to support their motor precision, balance, or athletic performance during tasks that demand high levels of coordination.

Brain Recovery and Cognitive Resilience

During times of cognitive recovery, such as after mental exhaustion or neurological strain, maintaining neurotransmitter balance can be a challenge. Tyrosine may help the body replenish dopamine and other critical compounds needed for brain performance. While it is not a treatment, some individuals include tyrosine in their routine to help maintain focus and mental resilience during recovery periods.

Customer-Reported Tyrosine Benefits

Tyrosine is widely recognized by users for its ability to support mental clarity, mood, focus, and emotional resilience. With an impressive average rating of 4.5 out of 5 stars across thousands of verified reviews, this amino acid has become a daily staple for many individuals looking to improve their cognitive performance, boost motivation, and support emotional well-being. While scientific research highlights Tyrosine's role as a precursor to important neurotransmitters, user feedback adds a powerful layer of real-world insight. The stories shared by reviewers consistently reflect noticeable shifts in energy, mood, and focus, especially during periods of mental fatigue, emotional stress, or cognitive strain. For those navigating challenges like low motivation, emotional flatness, or brain fog, Tyrosine appears to offer a gentle but meaningful sense of uplift and clarity.

Use Case Patterns Observed

Tyrosine is most commonly used by individuals seeking relief from low energy, emotional exhaustion, and lack of mental focus. Many reviewers describe turning to it as an alternative to traditional stimulants, or as a supplement to help them stay sharp and emotionally balanced in demanding situations. A large number of users mention struggles with long-standing brain fog, fatigue, and difficulty concentrating, or post-viral symptoms. Others incorporate Tyrosine as part of a broader wellness plan for mood support, recovery from alcohol dependence, or burnout due to stress. It is frequently used by professionals, students, and caregivers aiming to restore focus and motivation without the jittery effects of caffeine or prescription stimulants. Several users also describe using it during intense work periods, exam preparation, or while managing emotional lows from hormonal shifts or chronic stress.

Feedback Insights

The emotional tone of the reviews is both candid and heartfelt. Many users describe Tyrosine as life-changing, not because it creates a dramatic transformation overnight, but because it gradually lifts a mental fog they had come to accept as normal. Words like "clear," "motivated," and "focused" appear repeatedly, often paired with surprise at how quickly benefits were noticed. Several reviewers mention regaining interest in daily life, describing a shift from apathy or emotional flatness to a renewed sense of purpose and engagement. One user said it felt like their "pleasure receptors worked again," while another described finally "waking up with a smile."

Many express deep gratitude, especially those who had been struggling for years to find non-pharmaceutical options that felt safe and effective. A parent noted their teenager with attention challenges began smiling and dancing again, calling it a breakthrough in their home. Others noticed not just improved focus and emotional balance, but better sleep quality and a calmer response to stress. While a few experienced mild side effects like headaches, especially at higher doses, many of those cases were resolved with the addition of vitamin co-factors such as methylated B vitamins or adjustments to timing and dosage.

The emotional impact is clear: people feel more like themselves. For many, Tyrosine helped lift the heaviness that had been clouding their minds for years. As one reviewer simply put it, "This stuff gave me my life back."

Most Reported Benefits from Review Analysis

Tyrosine is a key amino acid known for its involvement in cognitive performance, mood regulation, and energy metabolism. Based on real-world feedback from thousands of users, Tyrosine consistently receives high praise, with an average customer rating of 4.5 out of 5 stars. Many individuals turn to Tyrosine to help overcome challenges like mental fatigue, lack of motivation, brain fog, and low mood. While the science behind Tyrosine supports its role as a precursor to dopamine and other important neurotransmitters, what stands out in user reviews is how often it makes a noticeable difference in their daily lives.

Our analysis focused on verified 4- and 5-star reviews that specifically mentioned benefits users experienced. The percentages shown below represent how frequently each benefit was cited in positive feedback. This approach offers valuable insights into how Tyrosine is most commonly experienced and where users feel it helps the most.

Tyrosine's Top Benefits Reported by Customers

Benefit	%	Explanation
Energy & fatigue reduction	29%	Boosts natural energy, helps reduce fatigue, and supports stamina throughout the day.
Focus & mental clarity	28%	Enhances mental sharpness, supports concentration, and reduces brain fog.
Mood & stress support	28%	Promotes emotional balance, supports a calmer response to stress, and lifts overall mood.
Motivation & productivity	8%	Encourages drive, supports consistent output, and helps users stay on task.

Benefit	%	Explanation
Thyroid & metabolic support	7%	Contributes to healthy thyroid function and may support metabolic balance.

How to Use This Table

This table provides a snapshot of what users most often report when taking Tyrosine. If you are exploring Tyrosine for similar wellness goals, such as reducing fatigue, improving focus, or lifting mood, this data can offer helpful perspective. The higher the percentage, the more frequently that benefit was observed by others with similar needs. As with all supplements, individual responses can vary, but this summary offers a useful guide to what real users have found most impactful. Consider starting with a thoughtful dose, tracking how you feel, and speaking with a healthcare provider if you have specific health conditions or are taking medications.

Tyrosine's wide range of reported benefits, combined with its consistently high ratings, suggests that it may be a valuable option for those looking to enhance mental performance, manage stress, and improve day-to-day motivation naturally.

Carnitine

Carnitine is a naturally occurring amino acid derivative that plays a critical role in energy production within your body. Often referred to as the "energy shuttle," carnitine facilitates the transport of fatty acids into the mitochondria, the powerhouse of cells, where they are oxidized to produce energy. While your body can synthesize carnitine from the amino acids lysine and methionine, supplementation can offer additional benefits, especially for individuals with increased energy demands or specific health conditions. Whether you're aiming to enhance athletic performance, support heart health, boost cognitive function, or promote weight management, carnitine provides a range of benefits that can significantly elevate your self-care routine and overall well-being.

Science-Informed Carnitine Benefits

Energy Production and Fat Utilization

One of the most well-known roles of carnitine is its support for mitochondrial energy generation. It acts as a transporter, moving fatty acids into mitochondria where they can be oxidized to generate ATP, the body's primary energy currency. This function becomes particularly important during prolonged physical exertion, when energy demand is elevated. By improving the efficiency of fat metabolism, carnitine may help reduce fatigue and promote greater endurance. This mechanism is of interest to those seeking additional energy support, especially in situations of physical or metabolic strain.

Support for Metabolic Health

Carnitine's involvement in fatty acid oxidation also has implications for metabolic function. By promoting the breakdown of fats, it supports a more efficient use of stored energy and may contribute to maintaining balanced lipid levels. Some research has explored carnitine's potential to influence triglyceride levels and overall metabolic parameters, making it a useful addition to a wellness plan focused on metabolic health and energy balance.

Physical Performance and Muscle Recovery

For individuals engaged in exercise, carnitine has been studied for its potential to improve performance and post-activity recovery. It may support endurance by delaying the onset of muscle fatigue and limiting the buildup of lactic acid during intense workouts. Some findings also suggest that it may help reduce the sensation of soreness following strenuous activity by supporting tissue recovery and oxidative balance. These properties are particularly appealing to athletes and physically active individuals looking for ways to enhance training outcomes and support recovery.

Cardiovascular Support

The heart relies heavily on fatty acid oxidation for energy, and carnitine is a key facilitator of that process. Its role in optimizing cardiac energy metabolism has drawn interest in the context of overall cardiovascular function. Some studies have observed that carnitine may influence lipid profiles by supporting healthy triglyceride levels and increasing beneficial HDL cholesterol. While not a treatment for cardiovascular conditions, these effects may contribute to general heart health and circulatory wellness when used as part of a comprehensive health strategy.

Cognitive Function and Brain Health

The brain is another high-demand organ where energy efficiency is vital. Acetyl-L-carnitine, a form of carnitine that crosses the blood–brain barrier, has been studied for its potential to support mental clarity, focus, and cognitive vitality. Through its role in mitochondrial energy production and antioxidant defense, carnitine may help protect neurons from oxidative stress and support healthy brain function as people age. While more research is needed, early findings suggest possible benefits for memory, attention, and overall cognitive resilience.

Weight and Body Composition Goals

Carnitine's ability to facilitate fat metabolism makes it a popular option among individuals pursuing body composition or weight management goals. By encouraging the body to use fat as an energy source more efficiently, it may complement diet and exercise efforts aimed at reducing body fat. Some users also report increased energy and reduced sluggishness while using carnitine as part of a structured wellness plan.

Reproductive Health and Cellular Energy

Carnitine has been studied for its impact on reproductive health, particularly in relation to energy production in reproductive cells. In men, carnitine supports the mitochondrial function of sperm cells, which may influence motility and overall vitality. For women, early research has explored carnitine's potential role in supporting ovarian cellular energy and hormonal balance. These properties reflect the broader importance of carnitine in tissues that require sustained energy supply for optimal function.

Customer-Reported Carnitine Benefits

Carnitine supplements continue to receive enthusiastic feedback from a wide range of users, particularly for their role in supporting energy, metabolism, recovery, and cognitive clarity. With a high average rating of 4.5 out of 5 stars, Carnitine has earned the trust of many individuals seeking a natural way to improve vitality and performance, both mentally and physically.

From those navigating chronic fatigue or thyroid-related exhaustion to fitness enthusiasts aiming for enhanced endurance and fat metabolism, thousands have turned to Carnitine and reported noticeable changes in how they feel and function. While individual experiences vary, there is a clear pattern of increased energy, improved exercise performance, and greater emotional and mental resilience. Many reviewers express deep gratitude for discovering this amino acid compound, describing the effects as uplifting, empowering, and sometimes even life-changing.

The following sections explore the most common real-world use cases and emotional reactions shared by verified buyers who found meaningful results with Carnitine.

Use Case Patterns Observed

Many individuals who turn to Carnitine do so with the goal of boosting energy, overcoming physical fatigue, or enhancing workout performance. A significant portion of reviewers mention using it in the context of structured exercise routines, often reporting better stamina, quicker recovery, and support with fat loss. Some use Carnitine as part of a larger weight management or supplement stack, frequently alongside CLA, green tea extract, or other metabolism-supportive compounds.

Another common pattern involves users dealing with thyroid-related fatigue or metabolic slowdown, including those with hypothyroidism or PCOS. In these cases, Carnitine was often chosen as a complementary tool to support energy production, reduce sluggishness, and improve physical activity levels. A number of users also shared their experiences using Carnitine to support cardiovascular wellness, cognitive clarity, and even reproductive health, particularly in the context of sperm quality or hormonal balance.

Several reviewers noted the importance of timing and dosage, often taking Carnitine first thing in the morning or before workouts on an empty stomach. Others emphasized that consistent use, rather than expecting overnight results, was key to seeing benefits.

Feedback Insights

The emotional tone in user reviews of Carnitine is often one of surprise, relief, and renewed hope. Many describe themselves as initially skeptical, unsure whether a supplement could make a noticeable difference. But after just a few days or weeks, users often found themselves more energized, motivated, and clear-headed, sometimes after years of struggling with exhaustion or stagnation.

One reviewer wrote, "I have fibromyalgia, MS, and hypothyroidism, and I'm very thankful this supplement works. It gives me the energy I need to get through the day." Another person with a long history of thyroid-related fatigue shared, "It's amazing. I feel like I have my life back." Many reflected on how Carnitine helped lift the mental fog, reduce that drained, heavy feeling, and reignite their drive to take action, clean the house, return to the gym, or simply feel more like themselves again.

For athletes and fitness-focused users, the tone often shifted to excitement and pride. One wrote, "I put 40 pounds on my bench press in just over a month. My recovery is way faster now. This stuff rocks." Another cyclist shared, "I usually ride 15 miles and this helped me pedal longer without my body giving out. The difference was impressive."

Some described emotional milestones that surprised even their doctors, including better fertility test results, thyroid numbers returning to normal range, or recovery from cardiac fatigue. These moments were often shared with deep gratitude, as one reviewer put it: "I was near hopeless after heart surgery, but Carnitine gave me my life back."

Even among those using it for more modest goals, like breaking through a weight loss plateau or curbing appetite, many emphasized the sense of empowerment that came from seeing consistent progress.

Most Reported Benefits from Review Analysis

Carnitine has become a popular supplement among individuals seeking natural ways to boost energy, enhance endurance, and support metabolic health. With an impressive overall customer rating of 4.5 out of 5 stars across thousands of reviews, it is widely praised for its ability to improve physical stamina, support weight management goals, and reduce the fatigue that often accompanies demanding lifestyles.

To better understand what users experience in real-world settings, we analyzed a large sample of verified 4- and 5-star reviews. We examined the specific benefits users most frequently mentioned and tallied those mentions to identify which outcomes stood out. The results provide a practical view into which wellness areas Carnitine may support most often, based on what users themselves have reported.

For example, if more than half of positive reviewers mentioned experiencing increased energy, it suggests that individuals seeking help with fatigue or low stamina might find similar value in this supplement.

The table below summarizes the top benefits reported by satisfied users.

Carnitine's Top Benefits Reported by Customers

Benefit	%	Explanation
Energy	54%	Reported to improve energy levels, reduce fatigue, and support daily vitality.
Weight Loss	22%	Frequently used as part of fat-loss regimens and credited with supporting weight reduction efforts.
Metabolism	9%	Helps support more efficient metabolic function and fat utilization.
Endurance	7%	Mentioned for boosting stamina and improving exercise performance.
Fatigue Relief	7%	Used by many to help combat tiredness and physical burnout.

How to Use This Table

This benefit table is designed to help you understand how Carnitine has been experienced by others, so you can make a more informed decision about whether it aligns with your wellness goals. A higher percentage means more users mentioned that specific outcome when sharing their positive results.

If you are seeking more sustained energy, greater physical endurance, or support for fat metabolism and weight management, these data suggest that you are not alone, and that Carnitine may be worth considering as part of your personal wellness strategy. Of course, individual responses can vary, and the best results are often seen when supplements are used consistently alongside healthy lifestyle practices.

These findings do not guarantee outcomes, but they reflect real-world patterns of use that may help guide your choices.

Arginine

Arginine, often hailed as a versatile and essential amino acid, plays a critical role in numerous physiological processes that contribute to your overall health and vitality. While your body can synthesize arginine from the amino acids lysine and methionine, supplementation can offer additional benefits, especially under conditions of stress, illness, or intense physical activity. Arginine is a precursor to nitric oxide, a powerful vasodilator that enhances blood flow and supports cardiovascular health. Beyond its role in nitric oxide production, arginine is involved in protein synthesis, immune function, hormone secretion, and the removal of ammonia from the body. Whether you're striving to boost athletic performance, support heart health, enhance immune resilience, promote wound healing, increase sexual drive, alleviate joint and chest pain, or reduce migraines, arginine provides a range of benefits that can significantly elevate your self-care routine and overall well-being.

Science-Informed Arginine Benefits

Cardiovascular Health

Arginine plays a vital role in cardiovascular support due to its function as a precursor to nitric oxide, a molecule that helps relax and widen blood vessels. This vasodilation effect promotes improved blood flow, supporting healthier circulation and helping to maintain blood pressure within a normal range. Enhanced circulation may also contribute to better vascular flexibility, which is important for heart and artery function. While more research is still ongoing, these mechanisms suggest potential benefits for individuals seeking to support overall cardiovascular health through improved blood flow and vessel integrity.

Athletic Performance

Supplemental arginine is often used by athletes and active individuals for its ability to support blood flow and oxygen delivery to working muscles. Improved circulation during physical exertion may help reduce the onset of fatigue and enhance stamina, making it easier to sustain performance in both strength and endurance activities. In addition, arginine contributes to protein synthesis, which plays a key role in muscle repair and recovery. These combined effects may offer supportive benefits for those looking to improve exercise efficiency and post-workout recovery.

Immune Support

Arginine contributes to the function of immune cells such as lymphocytes and macrophages. By supporting the activity and proliferation of these cells, arginine helps maintain a responsive immune system. Its potential anti-inflammatory properties also make it a valuable addition to routines focused on immune resilience. While it is not a replacement for medical treatments, arginine may serve as a supportive nutrient for those under physical stress or recovering from illness.

Wound Healing

Tissue repair and regeneration rely heavily on collagen production and efficient nutrient delivery, both of which are influenced by arginine. This amino acid supports the formation of collagen, the primary structural protein in skin and connective tissue, and promotes blood circulation to injured areas. These functions may contribute to a faster and more efficient healing process in minor wounds or post-surgical recovery. As part of a comprehensive wellness plan, Arginine may offer support in situations where wound healing is a concern.

Hormone Regulation

Arginine plays a role in stimulating the natural release of growth hormone, which is important for muscle development, metabolism, and cellular repair. It also supports insulin activity, potentially aiding the body's ability to regulate blood sugar levels. While not intended to replace medications for hormone-related conditions, arginine may be considered a helpful nutrient for those focused on supporting metabolic balance and hormone signaling.

Metabolic Function

The metabolism of protein in the body produces ammonia, a compound that must be safely removed. Arginine supports this detoxification process by facilitating the conversion of ammonia into urea, which is then excreted through the kidneys. This contributes to metabolic efficiency and may offer supportive benefits for liver health and the body's overall detoxification pathways.

Sexual Health

As a nitric oxide precursor, arginine helps facilitate healthy blood flow, including to areas involved in sexual function. Some individuals use it to support sexual wellness, including libido and arousal. Its circulation-enhancing effects have been studied in relation to male performance and erectile function, though responses can vary. In women, increased blood flow may also support arousal and sexual satisfaction. While not a medical treatment, arginine is sometimes explored as part of a natural approach to enhancing intimacy and reproductive wellness.

Pain Management

Through its potential to support circulation and reduce inflammatory responses, arginine may play a role in easing discomfort related to certain types of pain. Some individuals have explored its use for joint pain, back tension, or vascular discomfort. Enhanced blood flow may contribute to greater tissue nourishment and comfort in these areas. These benefits are often reported when arginine is part of a broader plan that includes lifestyle and physical care.

Migraine Relief

Migraine episodes are often linked to vascular changes and inflammatory responses in the brain. Arginine's ability to support healthy blood vessel function has made it of interest for those looking to manage the frequency or severity of vascular headaches. While research is still emerging in this area, its circulatory support may be one mechanism through which individuals experience relief as part of their wellness routine.

Customer-Reported Arginine Benefits

With a 4.3 out of 5 average rating across thousands of reviews, Arginine has earned a strong reputation among those seeking greater energy, circulation, and performance. While this amino acid is well-known for its role in nitric oxide production, the most compelling insights come directly from users who describe how it fits into their daily routines, whether to support stamina, vitality, libido, or overall cardiovascular well-being. From fitness enthusiasts and older adults to individuals managing blood flow concerns or energy dips, Arginine continues to resonate with a wide range of people looking to feel stronger and more alive. The following analysis captures the most common patterns in how real customers are using Arginine and what they are experiencing as a result.

Use Case Patterns Observed

Arginine is widely used by individuals seeking support for cardiovascular health, exercise performance, and male vitality. Many users begin supplementation to help with blood flow, vascularity, and nitric oxide production, often motivated by goals related to stamina, libido, or managing age-related changes. A large number of reviews came from men over 40 aiming to restore youthful energy, address erectile function challenges, or enhance muscle pump during workouts. Additionally, some users reported benefits in recovery from fatigue, workout endurance, and blood pressure support. A smaller but meaningful group used it for migraine relief, improved circulation, or as part of a natural wellness approach post-radiation, post-menopause, or during sedentary lifestyle transitions. Others incorporated it alongside citrulline, beetroot, or CoQ10 for synergistic effects.

Feedback Insights

Reviewers frequently described Arginine as a noticeable and empowering addition to their daily health routine. One mid-50s user noted, "This product gave me all-day energy… after a 10-hour day, I still had energy to do things around the house." Many emphasized the increased vascularity and stamina, with several calling out the visible "vein pump" during workouts as confirmation that the supplement was working. One user compared it to "feeling 25 again, in the gym and the bedroom," while another shared that Arginine gave him "the confidence to stop worrying and enjoy intimacy again."

Others highlighted emotional relief from discovering a non-prescription option that worked for them. "I don't have to worry about expensive prescriptions anymore," said one man after regaining erectile function. A female reviewer shared that it "felt like a biochemical war was raging on" as her gout symptoms rapidly improved with Arginine supplementation, describing a return to mobility she hadn't experienced in days.

Even skeptics became believers: "At first, I thought it was placebo, but then my partner commented without me saying anything," wrote one reviewer. Another mentioned, "After two weeks, I didn't just see results; I felt them. My drive came back, and I've been feeling more like myself."

While a few users noted side effects such as mild digestive discomfort or sensitivity due to low blood pressure, the majority found Arginine to be energizing, revitalizing, and confidence-boosting, especially when taken consistently. The most common sentiments were increased vitality, restored confidence, and the powerful feeling of being "back in control" of their health and performance.

Most Reported Benefits from Review Analysis

Arginine has become a popular choice among those looking to support cardiovascular wellness, circulation, and energy. With an average customer rating of 4.3 out of 5 across thousands of reviews, users often describe meaningful improvements in blood flow, stamina, nitric oxide levels, and overall vitality. Our review analysis focuses on the most frequently mentioned benefits reported by satisfied customers.

The percentages shown below represent how often each benefit was cited in positive reviews. A higher percentage means that more users experienced that benefit, suggesting a stronger likelihood of seeing similar effects if you share related wellness goals.

For instance, if 39% of positive reviewers reported increased energy, that indicates a common and consistent result experienced by those who used Arginine for that purpose.

Arginine's Top Benefits Reported by Customers

Benefit	%	Explanation
Energy	39%	Boosts overall energy, helps reduce fatigue, and promotes stamina.
Sexual Health & Performance	19%	Supports libido, healthy blood flow, and physical performance.
Blood Pressure	15%	Helps support healthy blood pressure by promoting vascular relaxation.
Nitric Oxide	11%	Enhances nitric oxide production to aid circulation and vascular function.
Circulation	8%	Improves overall blood flow and supports healthy vascular response.

How to Use This Table

This table provides a snapshot of what users most commonly report when taking Arginine. If your goals align with the benefits listed above, such as improved energy, circulation, or sexual vitality, you may find Arginine to be a helpful addition to your wellness routine. While individual results vary, these patterns reflect common themes across thousands of real-world experiences.

Keep in mind that consistency matters. Many users reported stronger benefits after taking Arginine daily for several weeks. As with any supplement, results may depend on dosage, timing, and how well it fits into your broader health strategy.

Serine

Serine is a non-essential amino acid, meaning your body can synthesize it naturally. Despite its classification as non-essential, serine plays a pivotal role in various physiological processes that are crucial for maintaining optimal health and well-being. As a building block of proteins, serine is integral to muscle development, enzyme function, and cellular structure. Beyond its structural role, serine is involved in the synthesis of other amino acids, neurotransmitters, and essential biomolecules like phospholipids, which are vital for cell membrane integrity. Whether you're aiming to enhance cognitive function, support skin health, improve metabolic processes, bolster immune resilience, or promote overall cellular health, serine supplementation can offer significant benefits. By understanding the multifaceted roles of serine, you can effectively incorporate it into your self-care routine to achieve a balanced and healthy lifestyle.

Science-Informed Serine Benefits

Cognitive Health

Serine contributes directly to brain health by acting as a precursor to important neurotransmitters, including dopamine and serotonin. These neurotransmitters help regulate mood, memory, and cognition. Serine also participates in the formation of phosphatidylserine, a key phospholipid in brain cell membranes that supports communication between neurons. By contributing to neurotransmission and protecting neural tissue from oxidative stress, serine helps sustain cognitive clarity and long-term brain resilience.

Mental Well-Being

Because of its role in neurotransmitter production, serine supports mental focus and emotional balance. It is often studied for its influence on psychological wellness, particularly for its ability to promote calmness and improve clarity of thought. People under chronic stress or those managing mental fatigue may benefit from consistent serine intake, which helps the nervous system adapt and recover from ongoing cognitive demands.

Skin Health

Serine is a key building block of ceramides, which are lipids that protect the skin's barrier and help retain moisture. By supporting ceramide production, serine contributes to skin hydration, elasticity, and overall resilience. It may be particularly beneficial for those experiencing dryness, irritation, or sensitivity. Serine also plays a part in cell regeneration, supporting the repair of minor skin damage and promoting healthy skin turnover.

Metabolic Function

In metabolic pathways, serine contributes to glucose regulation and energy production. It aids in the conversion of carbohydrates into usable energy and participates in the synthesis of other amino acids such as glycine and cysteine, which are vital for metabolic processes. This metabolic support may be especially relevant for individuals looking to maintain consistent energy levels throughout the day.

Immune Support

Serine plays a supportive role in immune cell proliferation and immune signaling. It helps maintain a balanced immune response by contributing to the building blocks required for antibody formation and lymphocyte activity. Additionally, serine has been noted for its role in modulating inflammatory pathways, helping the body maintain an appropriate response to environmental and internal stressors.

Cellular Health

At the cellular level, serine is indispensable. It contributes to the synthesis of phospholipids, which form the structural basis of all cell membranes. It also supports nucleotide synthesis, which is necessary for DNA and RNA production. These functions are vital for cellular replication, repair, and the maintenance of genetic integrity, processes that underpin tissue health, wound healing, and healthy aging.

Muscle Maintenance

Serine supports protein synthesis, which is key to muscle development and recovery. It also participates in the regeneration of muscle fibers after physical exertion or minor injury. As a contributor to endurance and post-exercise recovery, serine may be useful for active individuals or those engaged in physical rehabilitation, helping the body maintain muscle strength and reduce fatigue over time.

Customer-Reported Serine benefits

With an impressive average rating of 4.5 out of 5 stars, serine has captured the attention of individuals seeking improved cognitive clarity, stress resilience, and sleep support. Our in-depth analysis of real-world customer reviews reveals how people are using this amino acid to support both brain function and emotional well-being. Many users report meaningful changes in areas like mental sharpness, memory, sleep quality, and mood balance, often after struggling with persistent brain fog, sleep disruption, or stress overload.

These firsthand experiences offer valuable insights into how serine may fit into a self-care routine, especially for those navigating age-related cognitive changes, attention difficulties, emotional fatigue, or chronic stress. The following summary reflects common patterns observed across hundreds of reviews from diverse users, including older adults, working professionals, students, and caregivers.

Use Case Patterns Observed

Serine supplementation is most commonly used by individuals seeking to improve cognitive clarity, reduce mental fatigue, support sleep quality, and manage stress. Many users report turning to serine after struggling with brain fog, memory lapses, and emotional exhaustion, particularly in high-stress environments or during periods of hormonal or age-related cognitive decline. Several reviews come from people managing chronic stress, anxiety, or sleep disruption, while others focus on mental focus and productivity, especially in academic or professional settings. A number of older adults also report using serine to maintain cognitive sharpness and preserve memory as they age. In addition, caregivers and individuals dealing with neurodegenerative conditions like Parkinson's or early-stage Alzheimer's have expressed interest in serine for its potential role in supporting brain resilience.

Some users take serine as part of a broader stack that includes nootropics, magnesium, or sleep support supplements. Others discovered it through personal research, biohacking communities, or recommendations from integrative healthcare providers. A smaller but notable group includes parents administering serine to teenagers with attention-related challenges, as well as individuals who were dissatisfied with or unable to tolerate prescription sleep or anxiety medications. This diversity in use cases highlights serine's appeal across age groups, cognitive needs, and emotional wellness goals.

Feedback Insights

The emotional tone of the reviews reflects a deep sense of gratitude and personal transformation. Many users describe the impact of serine in vivid and heartfelt terms, expressing amazement at how it helped them "wake up refreshed," "feel sharp again," or "calm down without sedation." Words like "life-changing," "blessing," and "miraculous" are used repeatedly, especially among those who had previously spent years searching for solutions to sleep disruption or mental fog. One woman with chronic cortisol-related insomnia reported finally sleeping through the night and waking without dread or depression, experiences she had nearly given up on. Others shared that their mood stabilized, their thoughts became clearer, and long-lost cognitive sharpness returned "as if a light had turned back on."

Older adults frequently noted feeling more like themselves again, with improved word recall and faster mental response times. Several reviewers referenced feeling "15 years younger," "brighter," and "clear-headed," even after decades of cognitive decline. For people managing attention or memory issues, serine brought a sense of control and renewed confidence. Many remarked on how it helped them stay present and productive at work or in social settings, reducing feelings of overwhelm or forgetfulness.

Sleep was another standout theme. Reviewers spoke of deep, uninterrupted rest and vivid dreams, often contrasting serine with other solutions that either didn't work or came with side effects. Rather than feeling sedated, users described a calm return to natural rhythms. A number of people also reported reduced stress reactivity during the day and greater emotional resilience under pressure. Even among those who were initially skeptical or slow to notice results, a consistent pattern emerged: the longer serine was used, the more noticeable the benefits became, especially in sleep quality, mental clarity, and stress response.

Most Reported Benefits from Review Analysis

Customer reviews for serine reflect strong satisfaction across a range of cognitive and emotional wellness goals. With an average rating of 4.5 out of 5 stars, users frequently highlight improvements in sleep, memory, focus, and stress resilience. Many describe feeling more mentally clear, emotionally balanced, and better able to manage daily demands.

Our analysis below summarizes the top five benefits most often cited in positive reviews. The percentages reflect how frequently each benefit was mentioned across thousands of user reports. A higher percentage suggests a more common experience among users with similar wellness goals.

For example, if 41% of users reported better sleep, it suggests that restful sleep and relaxation are among the most likely benefits observed by those who chose to supplement with serine.

Serine's Top Benefits Reported by Customers

Benefit	%	Explanation
Sleep	41%	Aids in restful sleep and helps reduce nighttime awakenings. Many users report waking up feeling more refreshed and energized.
Memory	31%	Supports memory retention and recall, especially in individuals experiencing age-related or stress-related forgetfulness.
Focus	14%	Enhances mental clarity and processing speed, helping users stay attentive and on task throughout the day.

Benefit	%	Explanation
Brain Health	7%	Promotes overall cognitive resilience and neurological function, often used as part of long-term brain support routines.
Stress	6%	Helps reduce feelings of mental overwhelm and promotes a sense of emotional steadiness without drowsiness.

How to Use This Table

This benefit breakdown offers a practical starting point if you are considering serine as part of your wellness routine. If your primary goals include better sleep, sharper memory, or improved focus, the patterns above may help guide your expectations. However, individual results can vary depending on your body's unique needs and how consistently the supplement is used.

Many users report that noticeable effects develop gradually over the first few weeks. Some feel changes in sleep or mood within days, while others observe steady cognitive improvements over time. Consistent use, proper timing, and pairing serine with other supportive habits, like stress reduction and a balanced diet, can enhance your experience.

By reviewing what thousands of people have shared, you can make more informed, confident decisions about whether serine aligns with your personal wellness goals.

L-Theanine

L-Theanine is a naturally occurring amino acid most commonly found in green tea leaves (Camellia sinensis). Unlike many other amino acids, L-theanine is capable of crossing the blood-brain barrier, allowing it to influence brain activity directly. It has been widely studied for its potential to promote calmness, enhance focus, and support mental clarity, making it a popular choice for individuals seeking to manage stress and support cognitive performance.

While the body does not require L-theanine as an essential nutrient, research suggests it may offer several functional benefits when used as a dietary supplement. These include its influence on brain wave activity, neurotransmitter levels, and relaxation response, all without inducing drowsiness. Below are several areas where scientific studies have explored the potential supportive roles of L-theanine.

Science-Informed L-Theanine Benefits

Stress Support and Relaxation

L-Theanine has been shown to support the brain's production of alpha waves, which are associated with relaxed yet alert mental states. Unlike many calming agents, it does not appear to cause sedation, making it well-suited for use during the day. Some studies suggest that L-theanine may influence levels of cortisol, a hormone associated with the body's stress response, thereby helping to ease stress and support a more balanced mood.

Focus and Cognitive Function

Research indicates that L-theanine may enhance attention and focus, particularly when consumed alongside caffeine. This combination has been studied for its potential to promote sustained concentration and reduce mental fatigue. L-theanine on its own may also support working memory and mental clarity by influencing neurotransmitters involved in cognition, such as dopamine and serotonin.

Sleep Quality

Although L-theanine is not a sedative, it may improve sleep by helping to calm the mind before bedtime. By promoting relaxation and reducing mental tension, it may help individuals fall asleep more easily and experience more restful sleep. Several studies suggest that regular supplementation may support improved sleep quality over time.

Immune System Support

Preliminary research suggests that L-theanine may support immune function by enhancing the activity of certain immune cells and modulating inflammatory processes. Its calming properties may also support immunity indirectly by helping to manage stress, which can have a negative impact on immune resilience when left unaddressed.

Cardiovascular Wellness

L-Theanine's ability to promote relaxation may contribute to cardiovascular support by helping to maintain already healthy blood pressure levels. Some small clinical trials have observed modest improvements in blood pressure response among individuals under stress, although more research is needed to confirm its long-term effects.

Emotional Balance and Mood

Through its influence on neurotransmitters such as serotonin and dopamine, L-theanine may support emotional regulation and promote a sense of well-being. Studies have explored its potential to help ease occasional feelings of anxiety and support balanced mood, particularly in individuals experiencing mental stress or overstimulation.

Brain Health and Neuroprotection

L-theanine has demonstrated antioxidant and neuroprotective properties in laboratory settings, with studies suggesting it may help protect brain cells from oxidative stress and support healthy neural function. While more research is needed, these early findings have prompted interest in its potential role in long-term brain health and age-related cognitive support.

Customer-Reported L-Theanine Benefits

L-Theanine has earned a strong reputation among users for promoting calm, clear-headed focus without sedation. With a high customer satisfaction rating of 4.6 out of 5, this naturally calming amino acid is especially appreciated for helping manage stress, ease anxious thoughts, improve sleep quality, and sharpen attention. Thousands of users describe it as a gentle but noticeable aid in navigating the mental strain of modern life, offering a sense of centeredness during times of pressure, fatigue, or emotional turbulence.

Use Case Patterns Observed

Most users turn to L-theanine for help with daily stress, racing thoughts, and mild to moderate anxiety, especially when traditional solutions have fallen short or caused unwanted side effects. Many reviewers began using it after hearing about its relaxing effects from medical professionals, natural health practitioners, or popular wellness advocates. It is commonly used during periods of intense work pressure, life changes, or mental fatigue. Others report using it for chronic stress, insomnia, overstimulation, or as a companion to caffeine to smooth out energy levels without jitteriness.

Another frequent pattern involves users managing long-standing anxiety or mood imbalances and seeking a natural way to feel more emotionally balanced. A significant number also mention incorporating L-theanine into their nighttime routines to quiet the mind and support more restful sleep. Some users take it alongside magnesium or calming teas, while others pair it with nootropics or adaptogens for additional support with focus and cognition.

Feedback Insights

The emotional impact of L-theanine shines through clearly in user reviews. Many describe it as "life changing," "calming without being sedating," or "a miracle amino acid." A large number of reviewers expressed genuine surprise at how quickly they felt the benefits, often within 30 minutes, and how consistent those effects were over time. For individuals who have struggled for years with anxiety, panic, or high cortisol, L-theanine brought what one person called "a long-forgotten calm." Others noted that it helped "bring their personality back," "quiet the storm of thoughts," and "feel like themselves again."

Sleep-related benefits are another powerful theme. Reviewers often share that L-theanine helped them fall asleep faster, stay asleep longer, and wake feeling more refreshed. One user who had been taking prescription sleep aids for years said it was the first time they felt "naturally sleepy" instead of drugged. Another described being able to sleep through thunderstorms for the first time in decades.

In the context of focus and mental clarity, many users describe a "zen-like alertness" or feeling "mentally sharper without being overstimulated." Several users with ADHD or attention difficulties report noticeable improvements in productivity and motivation. This is especially common among those combining L-theanine with caffeine, who appreciate the balanced, smooth energy it provides without the crash.

Overall, the tone across reviews is one of relief, gratitude, and empowerment. Many express a sense of hope, describing L-theanine as something they now rely on to stay centered, focused, and emotionally resilient.

Most Reported Benefits from Review Analysis

L-Theanine continues to earn high praise from users seeking a natural way to unwind, regain clarity, and improve their sleep. With an impressive 4.6 out of 5 average rating across thousands of reviews, this gentle amino acid is frequently described as both calming and mentally clarifying, without sedation or sluggishness. It is particularly appreciated by people navigating high-stress lifestyles, anxiety, or sleep challenges, and many describe it as a turning point in their wellness routines.

Our analysis of verified 4- and 5-star reviews identifies the top benefits most commonly mentioned by users. These percentages reflect how frequently each benefit was reported within positive feedback, offering a practical guide to what people tend to experience when using L-Theanine consistently.

For example, if 35% of reviews mentioned better sleep, that means over one in three users highlighted improvements in their ability to fall asleep or stay asleep. These numbers provide valuable insight into how this supplement supports real-world wellness goals.

L-Theanine's Top Benefits Reported by Customers

Benefit	%	Explanation
Sleep	35%	Enhances sleep quality, supports restful nights, and helps quiet the mind before bed.
Calm	21%	Induces a state of relaxed alertness, often described as feeling more emotionally balanced or at ease.
Anxiety	19%	Helps reduce anxious feelings and emotional overwhelm, often cited by those managing daily stress or past trauma.
Stress	13%	Promotes stress relief by encouraging a steady mood and more measured responses to pressure.
Focus	11%	Improves mental clarity and attention without overstimulation, often used as a caffeine companion or nootropic aid.

How to Use This Table

The percentages in this table are based on real-world feedback from verified users. While everyone's body responds differently, these patterns suggest what you might expect based on your specific needs. If your primary concern is sleep quality, for instance, you may find L-Theanine particularly helpful, since over one-third of users cited better rest as a top benefit.

Keep in mind that effects can vary depending on dosage, consistency, and personal health status. Some people report feeling results within an hour, while others notice gradual improvement over a few days or weeks. As always, it's important to listen to your body, track how you feel, and consult a healthcare professional if you have underlying concerns or are taking medications.

GABA

Gamma-Aminobutyric Acid (GABA) is a naturally occurring neurotransmitter that plays a crucial role in regulating brain activity. As the primary inhibitory neurotransmitter in the central nervous system, GABA helps to calm neuronal excitability, promoting relaxation and reducing stress levels. Unlike stimulatory neurotransmitters that heighten brain activity, GABA works to bring balance by slowing down overactive nerve signals. This calming effect makes it an essential component for mental well-being, supporting mood stability, stress management, and sleep quality. Whether you're looking to ease anxiety, improve focus, or enhance overall mental resilience, GABA offers a natural approach to achieving a sense of inner calm and balance. Understanding the benefits of GABA can help you incorporate it effectively into your wellness routine for optimal mental and emotional health.

Science-Informed GABA Benefits

Stress Regulation and Emotional Calm

GABA functions as a natural "brake" in the brain, helping to inhibit excessive neural firing that can result from overstimulation or chronic stress. By tempering excitatory neurotransmitters such as glutamate, GABA fosters a balanced state that many describe as calm yet clear-headed. This makes it an area of interest for those experiencing stress sensitivity or emotional tension in daily life. Emerging studies suggest that higher GABA activity may correlate with more balanced emotional responses and a greater ability to adapt to everyday stressors.

Support for Restorative Sleep

Healthy GABA levels are essential for promoting deep, uninterrupted sleep. As an inhibitory neurotransmitter, GABA facilitates the transition from wakefulness to rest by quieting mental activity and reducing the time it takes to fall asleep. Studies indicate that GABA levels tend to be lower in individuals experiencing sleep challenges. Supporting GABA function may therefore promote more consistent sleep cycles and enhance overall sleep quality without causing sedation during waking hours.

Mood Balance and Mental Well-Being

GABA plays a stabilizing role in the brain's emotional centers by helping to regulate excessive neural activity. This contributes to a more even, centered mood and supports emotional resilience over time. Research has explored GABA's involvement in the brain's ability to manage emotional fluctuations and respond to internal or external challenges with composure. This makes GABA particularly relevant for individuals seeking to promote steadier mental states and improved emotional balance.

Clarity, Focus, and Mental Efficiency

Although GABA is most recognized for its calming properties, its role in maintaining neural balance also influences cognitive function. By reducing mental noise and overstimulation, GABA may support clearer thinking and sustained concentration. A balanced neural environment often enables better working memory, learning, and task performance, particularly in situations where distractions or internal restlessness might otherwise interfere.

Physical Relaxation and Muscular Ease

GABA's influence is not limited to the brain. It also extends to the body's motor control systems, where it helps regulate muscle tone. Research suggests that supporting GABA activity may contribute to reduced physical tension, including muscular tightness related to stress. This potential muscle-calming effect has made GABA a focus of interest for those looking to support physical comfort and relaxation throughout the body.

Nervous System and Cardiovascular Regulation

The sympathetic nervous system, which governs the body's stress response, can affect cardiovascular function when activated too frequently. GABA helps temper this activity, promoting a more relaxed state that may have a secondary impact on heart rate and blood pressure regulation. Some studies have explored the relationship between GABA activity and cardiovascular health, particularly in relation to stress-induced changes in autonomic balance.

Long-Term Neurological Support

Maintaining proper levels of GABA is important for protecting neurons against excitotoxicity, a condition where nerve cells become damaged due to overstimulation. This regulatory function supports overall brain health and may contribute to long-term cognitive resilience. Preliminary studies suggest that balanced GABA signaling may play a role in supporting healthy aging and brain function across the lifespan.

Customer-Reported GABA Benefits

GABA (Gamma-Aminobutyric Acid) has long been known in neuroscience as a key inhibitory neurotransmitter involved in calming the nervous system. For people living with high levels of stress, emotional reactivity, or sleep challenges, the search for balance often leads them to natural supplements like GABA. In our review analysis, we found that customers consistently turn to GABA in moments of emotional strain, seeking relief not only from mental tension, but also from the physical symptoms that often accompany it.

With an average rating of 4.4 out of 5 stars across thousands of verified reviews, users describe GABA as a supportive ally in cultivating calm, easing stress, and improving sleep. Many express initial skepticism, often rooted in years of trying conventional medications or feeling let down by other solutions, only to find themselves genuinely surprised by the results. For some, GABA became the first supplement that made a noticeable difference in both their mind and body.

Use Case Patterns Observed

The most common reason customers choose GABA is to address persistent anxiety, racing thoughts, or emotional tension that interferes with daily life. Many individuals report turning to it after struggling with prescription medications, especially when seeking a non-habit-forming option for emotional support. It is frequently used as a daily supplement by those managing generalized anxiety, panic episodes, or emotional overwhelm.

Another major use case is sleep improvement. Customers experiencing insomnia, especially those whose sleep troubles stem from overactive thoughts or nighttime anxiety, often describe GABA as helpful for settling the mind before bed. Several also mention pairing GABA with magnesium or melatonin to create a more complete evening routine.

Other patterns include people using GABA to support emotional regulation in high-stress environments, such as caregiving, shift work, or parenting. A notable group of reviewers mention combining GABA with L-theanine or other amino acids for a more personalized mood support stack. Lastly, some users report benefits related to physical symptoms such as muscle tension or mild pain, especially when stress contributes to their discomfort.

Feedback Insights

Across the board, reviewers describe their experience with GABA using language that reflects relief, gratitude, and emotional release. One user, who had spent years cycling through medications, shared that after just a few weeks on GABA, they felt like "the person I was always meant to be." Another said they could finally "stand being in their own skin," a sentiment echoed by many who felt GABA helped soften years of internal pressure.

For those dealing with anxiety, reviews frequently mention a subtle but meaningful shift. Rather than feeling sedated or disconnected, users report feeling grounded, calm, and mentally clearer. One reviewer noted that they didn't even realize how tense they had been until they experienced what it felt like to relax. Several reviews describe the first few days of use as transformational. Some users even said they felt emotional just realizing they could function without panic for the first time in years.

Sleep-related feedback is also strong, with users appreciating how GABA helped them fall asleep more easily and sleep more deeply without morning grogginess. One person described it as "taking the edge off the noise in my head," allowing their brain to finally rest. Others reported waking up feeling refreshed for the first time in a long time.

Even among skeptics, the change was sometimes dramatic. Many reviewers wrote that they "weren't expecting much" but were surprised by how quickly they noticed results, especially when taken consistently. Emotional phrases like "life saver," "my calm in chaos," and "a godsend" appear in numerous accounts, especially from those who had previously felt emotionally stuck or overwhelmed.

While not every user experienced the same results, and some noted mild tingling or temporary side effects, the majority expressed that GABA played an important role in helping them regain a sense of control, clarity, and ease in daily life.

Most Reported Benefits from Review Analysis

To better understand what users are actually experiencing, we conducted a deep analysis of verified customer reviews, focusing on the benefits most frequently mentioned by satisfied users. The table below reflects the distribution of reported benefits across thousands of positive experiences. While individual results always vary, a higher percentage suggests a more consistent pattern of benefit shared by others.

For example, 43% of reviewers specifically mentioned noticeable improvements in sleep, suggesting that if restful sleep is your goal, GABA may be especially worth exploring. Likewise, its calming effect and anxiety-reducing qualities were commonly cited, painting a picture of a supplement that many users turn to for emotional balance, better rest, and day-to-day stress relief.

Below is a summary table of GABA's top benefits as reported by customers:

Benefit	%	Explanation
Sleep	43%	Supports restful, uninterrupted sleep and may help reduce nighttime waking or difficulty falling asleep.
Anxiety	20%	Eases anxious feelings and promotes a sense of emotional calm during stressful situations.
Calm	20%	Encourages relaxation throughout the day, helping users feel more grounded and less reactive.
Stress	10%	Assists in managing daily stress and supports resilience during mentally or emotionally demanding periods.
Mood	8%	Contributes to a more stable and positive emotional state, often described as a sense of ease or lightness.

How to Use This Guide

If you are considering GABA for sleep support, emotional regulation, or help with everyday stress, these user-reported insights provide a practical starting point. The percentages above reflect how often each benefit was mentioned in real-world experiences, not a guarantee of outcome. However, they offer a clear view of how others are incorporating GABA into their wellness routines, and what results they most often describe.

It is also worth noting that many users reported multiple benefits at once, with effects often becoming more noticeable after several days or weeks of consistent use. Whether taken to unwind in the evening, to support calm focus during the day, or to promote emotional steadiness over time, GABA's consistent praise from customers makes it a trusted option for those seeking natural nervous system support.

Taurine

Taurine is a conditionally essential amino acid, meaning the body can produce it in small amounts, but under conditions of illness, stress, or intense physical activity, demand may exceed the body's natural ability to synthesize it. Unlike most amino acids, taurine is not used to build proteins. Instead, it is found in free form in tissues throughout the body, particularly in the brain, heart, retina, and skeletal muscles, where it plays critical roles in cellular health and physiological regulation. Taurine's involvement in processes such as electrolyte balance, mitochondrial activity, and antioxidant defense makes it a versatile compound for supporting whole-body wellness.

Science-Informed Taurine Benefits

Cardiovascular Support

Taurine has been shown to support cardiovascular function by promoting healthy blood vessel tone and helping regulate blood pressure within normal ranges. It is involved in calcium signaling within heart muscle cells, which contributes to steady cardiac rhythms and efficient contractions. Additionally, taurine may help protect blood vessels and heart tissue from oxidative stress and maintain proper balance in sympathetic nervous system activity, supporting a more resilient cardiovascular system overall.

Physical Performance and Muscle Recovery

Athletes and physically active individuals often turn to taurine for its role in exercise metabolism. Taurine contributes to muscle contractility and cellular energy efficiency, which may support endurance and reduce perceived fatigue during strenuous activity.

Some evidence also suggests that taurine helps reduce exercise-induced oxidative stress and supports quicker post-workout recovery. These combined effects make taurine a valuable addition to performance and recovery routines.

Visual Health

The retina contains high concentrations of taurine, where it plays a key role in maintaining the structural integrity and function of photoreceptor cells. Research suggests that taurine helps support eye health by acting as an antioxidant and promoting cellular stability within the visual system. Its presence in the retina is believed to help preserve clarity and function as we age.

Neurological and Cognitive Function

In the nervous system, taurine contributes to balanced neurotransmission and cellular protection. It acts as a neuromodulator and may help buffer overexcitation in brain cells, supporting cognitive steadiness and neural resilience. Preclinical research also suggests taurine may support mitochondrial health and protect neurons from oxidative damage, making it an area of interest in brain aging and neuroprotection.

Liver Health and Detoxification Support

Taurine assists in the synthesis of bile salts, which are essential for the digestion and absorption of fats. By promoting efficient bile flow and supporting liver cell function, taurine plays a role in the body's natural detoxification pathways. Its antioxidant properties also help shield liver tissues from environmental or metabolic stressors, making it supportive of overall hepatic function.

Cellular Hydration and Electrolyte Balance

Taurine helps regulate the movement of key electrolytes like sodium, potassium, and calcium across cell membranes. This contributes to optimal hydration and helps maintain cellular stability during times of stress or exertion. For individuals managing hydration, taurine may help support a more balanced internal environment and reduce the impact of electrolyte fluctuations.

Antioxidant and Inflammatory Support

Taurine exhibits antioxidant properties by scavenging reactive oxygen species and supporting the activity of other antioxidant systems in the body. By helping to modulate oxidative stress and inflammation, taurine contributes to cellular longevity and systemic balance. This makes it a valuable nutrient for individuals seeking to support long-term health and reduce the burden of everyday oxidative exposure.

Customer-Reported Taurine Benefits

Taurine has long been recognized for its critical roles in cardiovascular function, neurological balance, and cellular health. While scientific literature outlines its physiological importance, perhaps the most striking insights come directly from users who have incorporated taurine into their daily lives. With an average customer satisfaction rating of 4.6 out of 5 stars, taurine is consistently praised for its impact on energy, focus, sleep, mood, and heart rhythm. To understand how this supplement is performing in real-world settings, we analyzed hundreds of verified 4- and 5-star reviews. What emerged was a compelling picture of taurine as a trusted tool for those seeking physical vitality, emotional resilience, and deeper rest.

Use Case Patterns Observed

Taurine is used by a diverse range of individuals for a variety of wellness goals. One of the most common patterns involves cardiovascular support, particularly for those managing arrhythmias, blood pressure concerns, or age-related heart issues. Many users turn to taurine after years of trying prescription medications, often in search of a natural solution to complement or replace their current approach.

Sleep support is another leading use case. People struggling with insomnia, shallow rest, or nighttime interruptions frequently report turning to taurine for help achieving deeper, more restorative sleep. Some take it in the evening alongside calming minerals or amino acids, while others use it to manage daytime energy dips or regulate sleep-wake rhythms.

Cognitive support also features prominently. Several reviewers mention taurine's calming effects on the nervous system, noting benefits for focus, mental clarity, and emotional steadiness. Individuals experiencing chronic stress, public speaking anxiety, or brain fog often include taurine as part of a broader support strategy.

Additionally, users with inflammation-related discomfort, including muscle tension, weather-related pain, or joint issues, describe taurine as a helpful part of their anti-inflammatory regimen. A smaller but notable group uses taurine to support eye health, tinnitus symptoms, or metabolic balance, citing improvements in vision, hearing comfort, or energy levels.

Feedback Insights

Many users describe discovering taurine "by accident" or "out of desperation," often after other solutions failed to deliver. Their reviews carry a tone of cautious hope that quickly turns to enthusiasm. "I feel ten years younger," one reviewer shared after adding taurine to their routine. Another exclaimed, "This supplement changed my life," describing how chronic pain, migraines, or erratic heart rhythms dramatically improved.

Emotional well-being and calmness are major themes. Users speak of going from reactive and overwhelmed to composed and balanced. One described taurine as helping them face anxiety-inducing situations "with a very calm head," while another noted feeling less emotionally triggered during periods of stress or fatigue. Several reported that they and their loved ones noticed a significant reduction in irritability and a newfound sense of ease.

Sleep improvements are frequently highlighted. People who had struggled for years with poor rest report waking up refreshed, staying asleep through the night, and no longer dreading bedtime. "Morning grogginess is gone," said one user, while another shared that their teenage son was easier to wake and in a better mood after starting taurine.

Others found support in unexpected ways. One reviewer reported that their tinnitus had faded dramatically. Another was surprised to find that taurine helped reduce barometric pressure-related migraines. In several cases, people expressed amazement that something so simple had provided relief when more complex or costly treatments had failed.

The overall tone across these reviews is one of quiet astonishment. Even when benefits unfolded gradually, users frequently expressed a strong sense of gratitude, and many committed to keeping taurine as a permanent part of their wellness toolkit.

Most Reported Benefits from Review Analysis

To better understand how taurine performs in real-world settings, we analyzed hundreds of verified customer reviews, focusing on the most frequently mentioned benefits by satisfied users. While individual experiences vary, these percentages reflect the most common patterns among those who felt taurine made a positive difference in their daily lives.

If, for instance, 28% of users specifically mention improved sleep, that suggests a high likelihood of seeing similar benefits if sleep support is your personal goal. Similarly, mentions of increased energy, calmness, or cardiovascular support help paint a fuller picture of how taurine is being used across a wide range of needs.

Below is a summary table of taurine's top reported benefits based on customer feedback:

Benefit	%	Explanation
Energy Support	28%	Users frequently report feeling more energized, less fatigued, and mentally sharper throughout the day. Many describe a boost in stamina, especially during periods of physical or emotional stress.
Sleep Quality	28%	A significant number of reviewers say taurine helps them relax and sleep more deeply, often noting reduced nighttime waking and easier transitions into restful sleep.
Sense of Calm	15%	Many users describe feeling emotionally steadier and less reactive. They often refer to a noticeable calming effect, especially during challenging or high-pressure moments.
Stress Relief	13%	Some reviewers report that taurine helps them feel more resilient during times of stress, supporting emotional balance without causing grogginess or sedation.

Benefit	%	Explanation
Cardiovascular Support	9%	Users concerned about heart rhythm, blood pressure, or general cardiovascular wellness often mention taurine as a helpful addition to their regimen.

How to Use This Guide

If you are exploring taurine to support a particular area of well-being, such as increasing your energy, sleeping more soundly, managing stress, or enhancing heart function, these user-reported benefits offer a valuable reference point. The percentages above are not guarantees of outcome, but they do show how often each benefit appears in positive reviews from real-world use.

Many people report experiencing multiple effects at once, with improvements becoming more noticeable after several days or weeks of consistent use. The reviews often describe taurine as subtle but steady, offering gentle support without disruption to daily life.

Whether you are looking to address a specific wellness goal or simply support your body's natural rhythms, taurine's consistently high rating and broad appeal suggest it may be a helpful and worthwhile addition to your routine.

D-Aspartic Acid

D-Aspartic Acid (DAA) is a naturally occurring amino acid that plays a crucial role in the synthesis and regulation of hormones, particularly testosterone. Unlike its counterpart L-aspartic acid, DAA exists in smaller quantities in the body but has garnered significant attention for its potential to enhance athletic performance, boost libido, and support overall hormonal balance. Predominantly found in the brain, testes, and pituitary gland, DAA is involved in the release and regulation of luteinizing hormone, which in turn stimulates testosterone production. Whether you're an athlete aiming to maximize your performance, someone seeking to improve fertility, or an individual striving for hormonal balance, D-aspartic acid offers a range of benefits that can significantly elevate your self-care regimen and overall well-being.

Science-Informed D-Aspartic Acid Benefits

Hormonal Support and Testosterone Regulation

D-Aspartic Acid (DAA) plays a central role in regulating hormone synthesis, especially in its influence on testosterone production. It acts on the hypothalamic-pituitary-gonadal axis by stimulating the release of luteinizing hormone (LH), which then signals the testes to produce testosterone. This makes DAA a topic of interest for those seeking to maintain hormonal balance, particularly among men with concerns about declining testosterone levels. While research into its long-term efficacy continues, short-term studies suggest that DAA may help support healthy testosterone dynamics, which can affect energy, strength, and reproductive health in some individuals.

Physical Performance and Recovery Support

Because testosterone is a key factor in muscle protein synthesis, DAA has gained attention for its potential to assist with athletic performance. Some users report improved strength, endurance, and exercise capacity, especially when DAA is combined with regular strength training and proper nutrition. DAA may also support post-exercise recovery by contributing to hormonal balance, which is involved in reducing muscular fatigue and supporting the repair process following intense physical activity.

Fertility and Reproductive Wellness

DAA is found in the testes and is believed to influence spermatogenesis, the process by which sperm are produced. Preliminary research has explored its possible effects on sperm count, motility, and quality, particularly in men with suboptimal fertility markers. By supporting testosterone and luteinizing hormone levels, DAA may offer support to those focused on male reproductive wellness. However, results can vary, and DAA is best approached as one of several tools within a broader fertility-supportive strategy.

Cognitive and Neurological Function

Although better known for its impact on reproductive hormones, DAA is also present in the central nervous system, where it contributes to neurotransmission. Some research and anecdotal reports suggest it may help promote mental clarity, concentration, and cognitive resilience, particularly in stressful or mentally demanding situations. Additionally, DAA may have a role in modulating neural activity that supports cognitive performance, though further research is needed to confirm these effects in broader populations.

Vitality and Emotional Well-Being

Balanced testosterone levels are often linked to improved mood, energy, and motivation. Through its support of hormone production, DAA may contribute indirectly to enhanced feelings of vitality and reduced fatigue. While individual results differ, some people describe an increase in drive, motivation, and general emotional steadiness after consistent use. These benefits are typically experienced when DAA is used in the context of overall health maintenance, including sleep, diet, and lifestyle factors.

Customer-Reported D-Aspartic Acid Benefits

With an average customer rating of 4.4 out of 5 stars, D-Aspartic Acid (DAA) is a popular supplement among individuals seeking to support hormonal health, improve vitality, and enhance overall physical performance. Many reviewers specifically report benefits in energy, libido, motivation, and focus, especially among men over 40 experiencing the effects of declining testosterone levels.

Our analysis of thousands of positive customer reviews highlights the benefits users mention most frequently. While everyone responds differently, patterns emerge when enough people report the same outcomes. The table below reflects these shared experiences, offering practical insight into how D-Aspartic Acid is being used in the real world.

Use Case Patterns Observed

The majority of users turn to D-Aspartic Acid for its potential impact on testosterone-related functions. Many reviewers are men over the age of 40 who have experienced a noticeable drop in vitality, energy, libido, or motivation. Some had confirmed low testosterone or low luteinizing hormone levels, and used DAA as part of a broader effort to support hormonal balance. A smaller but meaningful number of users included DAA in their fertility or conception plans, while others combined it with strength training, resistance workouts, or testosterone-focused supplement stacks.

Some reviewers use DAA after periods of inactivity, weight gain, or illness, hoping to "restart" their system and regain momentum. Others use it for cognitive clarity or mood support, particularly if they had been feeling unmotivated or mentally foggy. Though most users were men, a few women also reported noticeable increases in workout energy and sweat response.

Feedback Insights

The emotional language across reviews often reflects a deep sense of renewal. Many users describe feeling "like themselves again" or even "like they did in their twenties," especially in relation to physical energy, mental focus, and sexual vitality. Words like "clear-headed," "driven," "energized," and "motivated" appear repeatedly, suggesting that DAA is valued not just for its hormonal impact, but for the quality of life improvements that often follow.

Some reviewers noted a shift within just a few days, describing their first week on DAA as "eye-opening" or "life-changing." Several mentioned having more endurance during workouts, increased muscle tone, or the motivation to return to exercise after long breaks. Others reported improved libido and mood, with one user even sharing that "it helped override low-level depression" and made them feel emotionally steady for the first time in years. Users with fertility goals shared stories of successful conception shortly after starting DAA supplementation, adding a deeply personal dimension to the feedback.

At the same time, a few users cautioned that DAA is most effective when low testosterone is linked to low luteinizing hormone levels, and that it may be less impactful in other scenarios. This level of thoughtful reflection and research awareness adds credibility to the overall sentiment: when used appropriately, DAA appears to deliver meaningful improvements for many people seeking hormonal and vitality support.

Most Reported Benefits from Review Analysis

To better understand how D-Aspartic Acid (DAA) performs in real-world use, we analyzed thousands of verified customer reviews, focusing on the most commonly cited benefits among satisfied users. The table below highlights the most frequently reported effects based on positive feedback. While individual responses may vary, a higher percentage suggests a consistent trend in how users experience the supplement's impact.

For instance, 37 percent of users highlighted noticeable support for testosterone production, suggesting that individuals with similar goals may also find DAA helpful in supporting hormonal health and physical performance. Energy, libido, and strength-related benefits were also regularly mentioned, painting a picture of a supplement that many users turn to when looking to elevate vitality, improve stamina, and enhance their physical output.

Below is a summary table of D-Aspartic Acid's top benefits as reported by customers:

Benefit	%	Explanation
Testosterone Support	37%	Frequently mentioned for helping users feel more energized, focused, and physically vital. Many associate it with a renewed sense of drive and improved hormonal balance.

Benefit	%	Explanation
Energy Boost	33%	Users often describe feeling more alert and motivated, with better endurance during the day and in workouts.
Libido Enhancement	13%	Many report a noticeable increase in sexual drive and satisfaction, especially among those seeking greater vitality with age.
Athletic Performance	9%	Praised for helping users perform better during exercise, with more stamina and smoother recovery.
Strength Gains	8%	Cited for improving power and physical output, especially when paired with consistent training.

How to Use This Guide

If you are exploring D-Aspartic Acid to support testosterone, energy, or performance goals, this table can serve as a helpful reference point. The percentages reflect how often each benefit was mentioned by customers in verified reviews, rather than a guarantee of results. That said, the data provides a strong indication of which outcomes are most commonly experienced.

It is worth noting that many users report experiencing multiple benefits at once, and that consistent use over time appears to play a key role in the perceived effectiveness. Whether you are pursuing enhanced workout results, greater energy, or overall well-being, this guide offers a real-world perspective on what DAA is most known for among those who use it regularly.

Glutamine

Glutamine is a conditionally essential amino acid, meaning that while the body is capable of producing it under normal conditions, its demand can rise significantly during times of physiological stress. Situations such as intense physical exertion, illness, trauma, or surgery can create a temporary deficiency, making external sources of glutamine beneficial for maintaining optimal function.

As the most abundant amino acid in the bloodstream, glutamine plays a central role in many aspects of human health. It serves as a building block for proteins, a vital energy source for rapidly dividing cells, and a key player in maintaining gut and immune health. Its widespread presence and critical functions make it one of the most researched amino acids in the context of both clinical and athletic settings.

Whether you are focused on recovery, immunity, digestion, or mental clarity, glutamine's multifaceted roles allow it to support the body in adapting to challenges, repairing tissues, and maintaining internal balance.

Science-Informed Glutamine Benefits

Immune Function Support

Glutamine is essential for the function of key immune cells, including lymphocytes and macrophages. These cells rely on glutamine as a primary energy source to proliferate and perform their protective functions. During times of immune challenge, such as infection, injury, or post-surgical recovery, the body's glutamine reserves can be quickly depleted. Supplementation during such periods has been studied for its ability to help preserve immune competence and reduce complications related to immunosuppression or physical stress. While not a treatment for any medical condition, maintaining adequate glutamine levels may help support a more resilient immune response.

Digestive and Gut Health

The cells that line the gastrointestinal tract have some of the highest metabolic demands in the body, and glutamine serves as a preferred fuel source for these intestinal cells. By providing energy and structural support, glutamine helps maintain the integrity of the gut barrier, which is essential for proper nutrient absorption and protection against unwanted substances crossing into the bloodstream. In research settings, glutamine has been investigated for its role in maintaining gut function under stress, including during periods of illness, fasting, or gastrointestinal distress. Individuals concerned with digestive wellness often consider glutamine as part of a gut-supportive nutritional plan.

Muscle Recovery and Protein Metabolism

In the context of physical activity and exercise recovery, glutamine plays a vital role in muscle tissue maintenance. It is involved in protein synthesis, muscle glycogen replenishment, and the reduction of muscle protein breakdown following strenuous activity. These functions can support more efficient recovery and reduce the time needed to return to baseline performance. While glutamine is not a direct muscle-building agent, it is often valued for its ability to assist in the recovery process, particularly among athletes or individuals engaging in high-intensity training.

Cognitive Function and Neurotransmitter Balance

Glutamine serves as a precursor to glutamate, one of the most important neurotransmitters involved in brain function. It contributes to the regulation of mental clarity, focus, and memory. By helping to balance excitatory and inhibitory neurotransmitters in the brain, glutamine may also play a role in mitigating mental fatigue, especially during prolonged stress or intense mental activity. Although its effects on cognition are still being explored, many individuals report improved clarity and concentration when maintaining adequate glutamine intake during mentally demanding periods.

Cellular Energy and Metabolic Support

Glutamine contributes to energy production by feeding into metabolic pathways such as the tricarboxylic acid (TCA) cycle. It is especially important for cells that divide quickly, including those in the immune system and the gut. By supporting mitochondrial function and energy metabolism, glutamine helps maintain cellular resilience and promotes tissue repair. This makes it particularly relevant for individuals recovering from injury, illness, or surgical procedures, when energy demand is elevated.

Adaptation to Stress and Physical Recovery

In both physical and psychological stress states, the body requires additional glutamine to sustain tissue repair, immune activity, and energy production. Supplementation during recovery periods may help reduce the impact of stress-related catabolism, support tissue regeneration, and promote a sense of physical balance. While not intended to diagnose or treat any condition, glutamine is often included in wellness routines for individuals navigating recovery from surgery, overtraining, or high-stress environments.

Customer-Reported Glutamine Benefits

Glutamine has received consistent praise across thousands of reviews, earning a strong overall rating of 4.5 out of 5 stars. For many, it has become a staple in their wellness routine, not because it promises overnight change, but because its effects accumulate and become deeply noticeable over time. Customers turn to Glutamine for a wide range of reasons, including digestive support, reduced bloating, improved energy, enhanced recovery, and help with sugar cravings. While individual results vary, a clear pattern of meaningful impact emerges from the voices of everyday users who have integrated this amino acid into their lives and routines.

Use Case Patterns Observed

Most users begin taking Glutamine in response to persistent gut discomfort, such as bloating, cramping, or digestive sensitivity linked to IBS, leaky gut, or post-antibiotic imbalance. Many describe years of struggling with discomfort after meals, food-related fatigue, or inflammation that did not fully resolve through diet or medication alone. Others report adding Glutamine to address cravings for sugar or processed food, especially during periods of dietary change, weight management, or recovery from substance use.

A significant number of reviewers mention pairing Glutamine with a clean diet, regular exercise, or probiotics to support gut healing, metabolism, and energy levels. Some athletes and fitness enthusiasts also use it for post-exercise muscle recovery, while others rely on it during periods of stress, sleep disruption, or immune system strain. Notably, several individuals going through alcohol or sugar withdrawal report meaningful emotional and physical support while using Glutamine, particularly when other methods had failed.

Feedback Insights

The emotional tone in reviews is overwhelmingly positive, often describing Glutamine as a "game changer" or "life saver" after long-standing digestive or craving-related struggles. Many users express genuine relief and gratitude, especially those who had grown frustrated with recurring symptoms or ineffectiveness of other supplements. One user described the experience as "finally feeling normal after every meal," while another shared, "I thought nothing could fix my bloating but then I found this."

For those battling sugar addiction, the emotional shift was just as clear. One reviewer wrote, "For the first time, I wasn't obsessing over dessert," while another shared, "I didn't even realize I hadn't had a craving all day until I sat down and thought about it." These changes were often described not just as physical improvements, but as emotional victories that renewed a sense of control and optimism.

Several reviewers also mention subtle but noticeable increases in energy, reduced fatigue after eating, and better sleep, sometimes described as "finally sleeping through the night" or "waking up feeling rested." Others praised its ability to support recovery, with phrases like "bounced back faster after workouts" and "less soreness than usual."

Even among skeptical users or those with complex health histories, Glutamine was often described as "surprisingly effective," "worth sticking with," or "the missing piece." Many reflected on how quickly they noticed changes, sometimes within a few days, and how symptoms returned if they stopped taking it. This reinforced the perception of real impact and motivated many to remain consistent.

Most Reported Benefits from Review Analysis

L-Glutamine has earned a strong 4.5 out of 5 rating from thousands of reviewers, many of whom describe it as a simple yet transformative addition to their daily routine. While individual results vary, clear benefit patterns emerge when examining the most frequently cited outcomes across highly rated reviews. These patterns reveal what users experience most consistently when supplementing L-Glutamine, particularly in areas related to digestive comfort, gut integrity, and sustained energy.

Our analysis categorized and quantified the most commonly mentioned benefits based on review frequency. These figures reflect how often users reported a specific improvement in their experience. The higher the percentage, the more frequently that benefit was mentioned in positive reviews. While no supplement works the same for everyone, this data helps set realistic expectations and identify the areas where L-Glutamine may be most impactful.

L-Glutamine's Top Benefits Reported by Customers

Benefit	%	Explanation
Bloating	43%	Helps reduce bloating and digestive discomfort, particularly after meals.
Gut Health	19%	Supports a healthy gut environment and promotes intestinal repair.
Energy	17%	Contributes to stable energy levels and reduced post-meal fatigue.
Leaky Gut Support	13%	Aids in strengthening the gut lining and maintaining intestinal integrity.
Stomach Issues	8%	Helps improve overall digestion and stomach comfort.

How to Use This Table

These reported experiences highlight the areas where users most often felt improvement when taking L-Glutamine. For those dealing with bloating, fatigue, or digestive sensitivity, this supplement may offer valuable support as part of a broader wellness strategy.

This table does not guarantee individual results, but it offers a clear snapshot of how users commonly experience the benefits of L-Glutamine. If you are seeking support for bloating, digestion, or gut health, these percentages suggest you may have a higher likelihood of experiencing noticeable improvement in those areas. As always, consistent use and integration with a supportive lifestyle tend to produce the best outcomes over time.

Using Non-essential Amino Acids

Amino acid supplements offer a practical and science-informed way to support various aspects of health and wellness. Often categorized as "non-essential" because the body can usually synthesize them, certain amino acids may still become conditionally important, especially during periods of stress, physical exertion, or recovery. These supplements are available in capsules or powders and can be incorporated easily into your daily routine to support nutritional balance and specific wellness goals.

Convenient Capsule Format

Capsules are one of the most widely used delivery methods for amino acid supplements. They offer a consistent, pre-measured dose, which is ideal for maintaining regular intake. Their portability makes them easy to take on the go. For those who prefer alternatives to swallowing pills, many capsules can be opened and mixed into water, smoothies, or food. This flexibility allows for personalized use, especially when incorporating amino acids into a broader health regimen.

Starting Slowly: Dosage and Adjustment

If you are new to amino acid supplements, it is often recommended to begin with a smaller dose. This gradual approach allows you to monitor how your body responds before increasing to the full amount suggested on the product label. These standard guidelines are typically intended for general wellness support. However, for targeted needs, adjusting the dose under the guidance of a qualified practitioner can help align supplementation with your specific goals.

When to Take Amino Acids

The best time to take an amino acid supplement may vary depending on your reason for using it. For instance, if your goal is to support recovery or physical performance, you may find it helpful to take it before or after exercise. Others may prefer to take it in the morning for energy or in the evening to support rest and recovery. Be sure to review the product label for timing instructions and consult with a practitioner if you are unsure what works best for you.

With or Without Food

Amino acid supplements are generally well tolerated and can often be taken with or without food. Those with sensitive stomachs may benefit from taking them alongside meals to enhance digestion and reduce the likelihood of mild gastrointestinal discomfort. If preferred, some individuals may choose to take them on an empty stomach, especially if that timing aligns better with their routine or goals.

Safety and Precautions

While amino acid supplements are typically well tolerated when used as directed, it's important to consider the following precautions:

Existing Health Conditions: If you have a diagnosed medical condition or are taking prescription medications, consult your healthcare provider before starting any new supplement.

Pregnancy and Breastfeeding: Speak with a qualified professional to determine whether amino acid supplementation is appropriate during this time.

Dosage Limits: Avoid exceeding the recommended dosage unless directed by a practitioner. Even natural compounds can have unwanted effects if used in excess.

By starting gradually, following dosage recommendations, and aligning timing with your individual needs, amino acid supplements can be a thoughtful and effective addition to your health routine. For best results, pair their use with balanced nutrition, physical activity, and professional guidance when needed.

Amino Acids for Everyday Health Goals

Grounded in both scientific insights and real-world experiences, this section connects common wellness goals with specific amino acid supplements, helping you easily identify supportive options that others have found helpful. Each amino acid listed includes user-reported benefit percentages and explanatory notes based on feedback, allowing you to make informed and confident decisions.

Along with this real-world validation, each supplement is also backed by scientific research, highlighting key findings from studies that support its potential benefits.

Whether your goal is to support immune resilience, improve focus, manage stress, or increase daily energy, this guide is here to provide trustworthy, user-informed information. Use it as a practical reference to explore how amino acid supplementation may complement your wellness journey and contribute to overall vitality.

Cardiovascular Health

Arginine (15%) – Blood Pressure Support.

Supports healthy blood pressure by promoting nitric oxide production and encouraging vascular relaxation. Research has shown that arginine serves as a precursor to nitric oxide, which contributes to proper blood vessel tone and improved endothelial function.

Arginine (11%) – Nitric Oxide Enhancement.

Enhances nitric oxide levels to support circulation and cardiovascular performance. Studies link arginine supplementation with improved blood flow, making it a valuable nutrient for heart and vascular support.

Cognitive Health

Serine (31%) – Memory Support.

Promotes memory retention and cognitive clarity, particularly during mentally demanding tasks. Research indicates that serine plays a role in neurotransmitter production and neuronal communication, both essential for learning and recall.

Tyrosine (28%) – Focus and Clarity.

Supports mental alertness and reduces cognitive fatigue, especially under stress. Scientific studies confirm that tyrosine is a precursor to dopamine, which helps regulate attention, motivation, and overall cognitive performance.

Phenylalanine (16%) – Focus and Clarity.

Improves concentration by supporting neurotransmitter activity. Research shows that phenylalanine converts into tyrosine, fueling the production of brain chemicals involved in focus and mental sharpness.

NAC (12%) – Brain Fog Reduction.

Helps ease brain fog and supports sustained mental clarity. Studies show that NAC boosts glutathione levels in the brain, providing antioxidant protection and promoting cognitive resilience.

Digestive Health

Glutamine (43%) – Gut Health and Bloating Relief.

Helps relieve digestive discomfort and supports the intestinal lining, reducing bloating. Scientific research highlights glutamine's role as a primary nutrient for gut lining repair and digestive system integrity.

Glutamine (32%) – Leaky Gut and Intestinal Repair.

Supports gut barrier function in those experiencing symptoms of leaky gut. Studies indicate glutamine helps strengthen tight junctions and supports a healthy intestinal environment.

Energy and Fatigue

Carnitine (54%) – Energy and Fatigue Reduction.

Many users report feeling more energized and less fatigued with carnitine supplementation. Research shows that carnitine assists in transporting fatty acids into mitochondria, where they are converted into ATP, the body's primary energy source. This process supports both cellular energy production and physical performance.

Arginine (39%) – Energy Support.

Users frequently note improved stamina and vitality, especially during exercise or demanding tasks. Scientific studies confirm that arginine promotes vasodilation by increasing nitric oxide production, which may enhance circulation and nutrient delivery to muscles and tissues.

EAAs (35%) – Energy and Endurance.

Essential amino acids help maintain energy levels during sustained physical activity and support post-exercise recovery. Research indicates that EAAs are vital for protein synthesis and metabolic function, playing a central role in supporting energy metabolism.

D-Aspartic Acid (33%) – Hormonal Energy Support.

Some users report enhanced vitality and reduced fatigue, which may be linked to improved hormonal balance. Studies suggest that D-aspartic acid can influence the body's natural testosterone production, contributing to increased energy levels, particularly in men.

Tyrosine (29%) – Energy and Mental Alertness.

Supports both physical stamina and mental clarity, especially under stress. Scientific evidence shows that tyrosine serves as a precursor to key neurotransmitters like dopamine and norepinephrine, which are involved in alertness, motivation, and stress response.

Taurine (28%) – Cellular Energy Support.

Many users describe feeling less tired and more resilient when using taurine, particularly under physical or emotional stress. Research suggests taurine supports mitochondrial health and calcium regulation, which are essential for sustained energy.

Phenylalanine (27%) – Mental and Physical Energy.

Reported to enhance wakefulness and reduce feelings of sluggishness. Scientific studies show that phenylalanine converts into tyrosine, helping to fuel neurotransmitter activity that supports energy, mood, and focus.

Glutathione (22%) – Fatigue Reduction.

Some users feel more refreshed and better able to manage daily demands. Research shows that glutathione helps neutralize oxidative stress and supports mitochondrial efficiency, which may contribute to sustained energy levels throughout the day.

Immune Support

Lysine (56%) – Cold Sore and Viral Response Support.

Many users report fewer and less intense cold sore episodes when taking lysine consistently. Scientific studies suggest lysine may interfere with the replication process of the herpes simplex virus and support the body's natural immune defenses.

NAC (17%) – Immune Resilience.

Users frequently turn to NAC during times of stress or illness, reporting stronger immune resilience. Research shows NAC supports the production of glutathione, a vital antioxidant that aids immune cell function and the body's natural defense mechanisms.

Lysine (14%) – General Immune Support.

Beyond its role in cold sore prevention, users also rely on lysine to support broader immune health. Scientific research indicates lysine may help modulate immune response and reduce susceptibility to certain viral challenges.

Glutathione (10%) – Inflammation and Immune Balance.

Some users report fewer immune disruptions and improved general wellness with glutathione. Scientific evidence confirms its role as a master antioxidant that helps regulate inflammation and supports immune efficiency.

Metabolic Health

Carnitine (22%) – Fat Metabolism and Weight Support.

Many users seeking metabolic support report increased energy and enhanced fat utilization with carnitine. Scientific studies confirm carnitine's key role in transporting fatty acids into the mitochondria, where they are converted into energy, supporting both metabolism and physical performance.

Respiratory Support

NAC (21%) – Respiratory and Mucus Clearance.

Users managing occasional congestion or mild respiratory concerns often report easier breathing and improved airway comfort. Scientific studies support NAC's function as a mucolytic agent, which helps break down mucus and supports lung health through its antioxidant properties.

Skeletal & Muscular Health

BCAAs (40%) – Workout Support and Endurance.

Users commonly report improved training capacity and reduced fatigue during workouts. Scientific studies indicate that branched-chain amino acids, leucine, isoleucine, and valine, support muscle protein synthesis and may help minimize muscle breakdown during exercise.

EAAs (36%) – Strength and Recovery Support.

Athletes and active individuals often experience improved strength and faster recovery with essential amino acids. Research confirms that EAAs supply all nine essential building blocks needed to stimulate protein synthesis and reduce post-exercise soreness.

BCAAs (26%) – Support for Lean Muscle Gains.

Users focused on building lean mass often rely on BCAAs. Scientific findings show that leucine, in particular, activates the mTOR signaling pathway, which plays a central role in initiating muscle growth.

EAAs (20%) – Muscle Repair and Recovery.

Many users report quicker recovery and less discomfort after physical activity. Studies support that EAAs promote muscle tissue repair by providing the full spectrum of essential amino acids required for optimal recovery.

BCAAs (19%) – Recovery and Fatigue Reduction.

Those using BCAAs regularly report less soreness and shorter recovery time. Scientific evidence suggests they help reduce muscle protein breakdown and support quicker post-workout recovery, especially in resistance training.

Skin Health

Glutathione (40%) – Skin Tone and Radiance.

Users often describe brighter skin, reduced dark spots, and a more even complexion. Scientific studies suggest that glutathione supports skin health by helping regulate melanin production and protecting against oxidative stress.

Lysine (22%) – Skin Support and Clarity.

Many users report fewer breakouts and improved skin texture. Scientific research supports lysine's role in collagen formation and maintaining skin integrity, which can contribute to healthier-looking skin.

Restful Sleep

Glycine (85%) – Sleep Quality and Relaxation.

Many users report deeper, more restful sleep and an easier time winding down at night. Scientific research suggests that glycine may lower core body temperature and support the nervous system in preparing for sleep, which can contribute to more effective sleep cycles.

Tryptophan (55%) – Sleep Support.

Individuals experiencing occasional sleeplessness often find tryptophan helpful in falling and staying asleep. Studies indicate that tryptophan serves as a precursor to both serotonin and melatonin, which are involved in the regulation of healthy sleep patterns.

GABA (43%) – Sleep and Insomnia Relief.

Users commonly describe fewer nighttime awakenings and a more settled, calm rest. Scientific studies show that GABA is the brain's main calming neurotransmitter, helping reduce neural overactivity that can interfere with sleep.

Serine (41%) – Restful Sleep and Nervous System Support.

Some users note greater relaxation before bed and improved sleep continuity. Research suggests that serine supports neurotransmitter balance, which may play a role in regulating sleep and calming the nervous system.

Theanine (35%) – Deep Sleep and Mental Calm.

Many report smoother sleep onset and less nighttime anxiety. Scientific evidence shows that theanine supports alpha brainwave activity, associated with calm alertness and improved sleep readiness.

Taurine (28%) – Relaxation and Sleep Enhancement.

Users frequently mention better sleep quality and reduced restlessness. Research supports taurine's role in modulating GABA receptors and maintaining neural stability, which may aid in restful sleep.

Reproductive and Hormonal Support

Arginine (19%) – Sexual Health and Circulation.

Users often report improved physical responsiveness and sexual vitality. Scientific research shows that arginine promotes nitric oxide production, which helps support healthy blood flow and vascular function important for sexual health.

D-Aspartic Acid (13%) – Libido and Hormonal Support.

Some users experience increased sexual interest and improved hormonal balance. Scientific studies suggest that D-aspartic acid may play a role in regulating hormone signaling pathways, including testosterone production.

Stress Support

Phenylalanine (47%) – Mood and Emotional Support.

Many users report greater emotional steadiness and a brighter outlook. Scientific findings show that phenylalanine is converted into tyrosine, a precursor to dopamine and other neurotransmitters that influence mood.

Theanine (40%) – Calm Focus and Relaxation.

Individuals often describe a more relaxed mental state without sedation. Studies support that theanine increases alpha brainwave activity, which is associated with calmness and stress reduction.

GABA (40%) – Support for Nervous System Balance.

Users commonly note a decrease in feelings of nervousness and greater day-to-day calm. Scientific evidence shows that GABA helps regulate excitatory signals in the brain, promoting a more balanced emotional response.

Tyrosine (28%) – Stress Adaptation and Mental Clarity.

Many report improved focus and resilience in high-stress situations. Scientific research indicates that tyrosine helps replenish neurotransmitters that are depleted during stress, supporting clearer thinking and better emotional coping.

Tryptophan (27%) – Mood and Stress Regulation.

Users describe reduced tension and a more balanced emotional state. Scientific studies confirm that tryptophan supports serotonin production, which plays a key role in emotional regulation and stress response.

A Final Word: The Journey to Vibrant Health

As we conclude this exploration of Amino Acid Therapy, it's worth reflecting on the simplicity and potential of what you've discovered. The tools and insights in this book are designed to support your health naturally, fitting into the rhythms of daily life, whether you're looking to enhance your well-being, navigate health challenges, or simply feel your best more consistently.

Throughout this book, you've learned how amino acids play an essential role in supporting key functions in the body, from energy and mood to digestion, sleep, immune function, and more. This approach works in harmony with your body, aiming to nourish foundational systems rather than just managing symptoms. Whether your focus is boosting vitality, supporting emotional balance, or improving recovery, amino acids offer a practical, research-supported way to reinforce your health from the inside out.

One of the greatest strengths of this therapy is its accessibility. You don't need to follow complex regimens or make drastic changes to experience meaningful benefits. Instead, these supplements can integrate naturally into your routine, providing support that feels intuitive, sustainable, and aligned with your long-term wellness goals.

This book is more than a reference guide; it's a starting point for empowered self-care. With the tools now in your hands, you can move forward with greater clarity and confidence. You no longer have to guess what might work or rely solely on conventional options. You have a framework built on science, real-world experiences, and nature's own building blocks.

As you begin to apply what you've learned, remember that healing is a process. Progress often comes from small, consistent actions, not perfection. Listen to your body, adjust thoughtfully, and celebrate the improvements along the way. Every step you take is a signal to your body that you are ready for balance, strength, and renewal.

This journey is uniquely yours, but you are not alone. The *Medicine-Free, Illness-Free Series* is here to guide you, with additional volumes on Herbal Therapy, Mushroom Therapy, Animal Organ Therapy, the HOPED Protocol, Detoxification Therapy, Grounding Therapy, and more. Each book offers natural strategies to support lifelong health, rooted in practical wisdom and emerging research.

May this book serve as an encouraging companion on your wellness path. The ability to heal and thrive is already within you, and now, you have a roadmap to unlock it.

This book is part of a larger journey to natural healing. To explore more solutions or receive personalized guidance, visit AshiHealing.com.

About the Author

Dr. Forest Yin (Jie Yin) is a licensed acupuncturist, herbalist, and Doctor of Acupuncture and Oriental Medicine (DAOM). He serves as a professor and doctoral advisor at the University of East West Medicine (UEWM) and is the founder of Ashi Healing and Acupuncture Inc. With extensive experience in Traditional Chinese Medicine (TCM) and natural health, Dr. Yin integrates a wide range of holistic therapies, forming the foundation of *The Medicine-Free, Illness-Free Series.*

Before devoting his career fully to natural healing, Dr. Yin worked in the high-tech and financial sectors with both large corporations and fast-paced startups. These experiences gave him firsthand insight into the chronic stress and burnout common in modern life. Inspired to seek sustainable strategies for long-term wellness, he turned to the wisdom of nature and the depth of Chinese medicine.

Dr. Yin's clinical experience and ongoing research have helped shape practical wellness protocols that focus on balance, energy, and lifestyle-based health support. His work emphasizes simple, science-informed approaches that align with the body's natural rhythms and support overall resilience.

Driven by a mission to empower others, he created *The Medicine-Free, Illness-Free Series* to share accessible natural strategies that fit seamlessly into busy lives. His approach blends ancient healing principles with modern insight, helping people feel more energized, focused, and in tune with their long-term health goals.

Continue Your Wellness Journey

This book is just the beginning. True wellness is a lifelong journey, and you don't have to walk it alone. The Ashi Healing ecosystem is here to support you every step of the way with personalized guidance, nature-based solutions, and a shared mission: to help more people experience the benefits of natural health.

Personalized Virtual Consultation

If you're ready for expert guidance tailored to your specific needs, you can schedule a private virtual consultation with Dr. Forest Yin at AshiHealing.com. These one-on-one sessions offer a personalized supplement and herbal plan based on your current wellness goals, lifestyle, and health history, helping you create a sustainable path forward using time-tested, natural approaches.

In-Person Consultation and Acupuncture

If you're located in the San Francisco Bay Area, Dr. Yin also provides in-person consultations and acupuncture sessions at the University of East West Medicine (UEWM) campus in Sunnyvale, California, where he also teaches in the doctoral program for Traditional Chinese Medicine. This serene, professional setting offers a welcoming space for personalized care. All visits, virtual or in-person, can be scheduled through AshiHealing.com.

Supplement Recommendation Plans

Each wellness protocol discussed in this book has a corresponding supplement plan available on Fullscript, featuring practitioner-trusted, food-based formulas. These curated plans make it easy to take action without guesswork, offering clear, guided steps for nutritional support.

You can access them directly at:

https://us.fullscript.com/welcome/ashi-healing,

or simply start from AshiHealing.com.

Explore the Complete Book Series

This book is part of *The Medicine-Free, Illness-Free Series*, a 10-book collection designed to help you support your long-term health and vitality through natural methods. Each volume introduces a unique modality—from herbs and mushrooms to detoxification, grounding, amino acids, and more—so you can build your wellness path one step at a time.

Refer to the Series Overview chapter or visit AshiHealing.com to explore the full collection.

Support the Natural Health Movement

If this book has inspired you, and you believe more people should have access to clear, trustworthy information about natural health, consider supporting our mission.

The Ashi Healing Foundation *(AshiHealing.org)* is a nonprofit organization dedicated to public education, natural health awareness, and holistic wellness outreach. Your tax-deductible donation helps expand access to these tools and empowers more individuals to explore safe, evidence-informed approaches to well-being.

To contribute, visit AshiHealing.org and join the movement for a healthier, freer world.

Connect and Stay Inspired

Your healing journey doesn't end here.

Follow **Dr. Forest Yin** for more healing stories, tips, and inspiration:

Instagram, TikTok, YouTube, and X: @DrForestYin

Facebook: @DrForestYin1

LinkedIn: linkedin.com/in/forest-yin

Ready to Take the Next Step?

Scan the QR code below to visit AshiHealing.com, your starting point for virtual consultations, supplement plans, and more resources.

Your journey toward sustainable, natural wellness begins now.

Made in the USA
Monee, IL
08 November 2026

68007849R00121